Atlas of
DIABETES MELLITUS

Atlas of
DIABETES MELLITUS
Third Edition

Ian N Scobie MD FRCP

Consultant Endocrinologist
Medway Maritime Hospital
Gillingham, Kent
UK

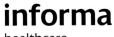

informa
healthcare

First published in the United Kingdom in 1998 by Parthenon Publishing
Third edition published in 2007 by Informa Healthcare, 4 Park Square, Milton Park, Abingdon, Oxon OX14 4RN.
Informa Healthcare is a trading division of Informa UK Ltd. Registered Office: 37/41 Mortimer Street, London W1T 3JH.
Registered in England and Wales Number 1072954.

Tel.: +44 (0)20 7017 6000
Fax: +44 (0)20 7017 6699
E-mail: info.medicine@tandf.co.uk
Website: www.informahealthcare.com

Second printing 2007

A CIP record for this book is available from the British Library.

Library of Congress Cataloging-in-Publication Data

Data available on application

ISBN10: 0-415-37649-1
ISBN13: 978-0-415-37649-5

Distributed in North and South America by

Taylor & Francis
6000 Broken Sound Parkway, NW, (Suite 300)
Boca Raton, FL 33487, USA

Within Continental USA
Tel.: 1(800)272 7737; Fax: 1(800)374 3401
Outside Continental USA
Tel.: (561)994 0555; Fax: (561)361 6018
E-mail: orders@crcpress.com

Distributed in the rest of the world by
Thomson Publishing Services
Cheriton House
North Way
Andover, Hampshire SP10 5BE, UK
Tel.: +44 (0)1264 332424
E-mail: tps.tandfsalesorder@thomson.com

Composition by Parthenon Publishing

Printed and bound in India by Replika Press Pvt. Ltd.

Contents

Foreword – *Robert A Rizza*   vii

Preface   ix

Acknowledgments   x

1.   Introduction   1

2.   Pathogenesis   9

3.   Treatment   33

4.   Treatment of children and adolescents with diabetes   59

5.   Diabetes and surgery   61

6.   Acute complications of diabetes   63

7.   Chronic complications of diabetes   69

8.   Diabetic dyslipidemia   109

9.   Diabetes and pregnancy   111

10. Living with diabetes   115

11. Future developments in diabetes   117

Index   121

Foreword

Diabetes mellitus is likely to become one of the most prevalent and economically important diseases of the 21st century largely owing to an increasing incidence of type 2 diabetes mellitus (DM) in the developed nations and many of the developing nations. Every physician will encounter a patient who has diabetes. Multiple factors, both environmental and genetic, contribute to the pathogenesis of the disease. Type 2 DM is particularly common in obese sedentary populations, while type 1 DM can have a dramatic onset and be a major therapeutic challenge.

Rarer conditions such as acromegaly, Cushing's disease and hemochromatosis may cause or exacerbate diabetes. If the hyperglycemia of diabetes is not adequately treated, potentially devastating micro- and macrovascular complications might ensue. It follows that all physicians need to be familiar with this condition and its array of complications and associations. However, owing to the sheer volume of information related to this area of medicine, it is difficult for the busy practitioner to keep up to date.

The third edition of Ian Scobie's *Atlas of Diabetes Mellitus*, building on the success of the two previous editions, goes a long way towards making this task easier and remains a testimonial to the fact that a picture is indeed worth at least a thousand words. This Atlas begins with a brief overview of the diagnosis, pathogenesis and treatment of diabetes with special reference to the complications of diabetes and the treatment of children and adolescents. Specific chapters cover diabetic dyslipidemia, diabetes and pregnancy and what it is like to live with this chronic condition. These, and other sections, set the stage for the multitude of highly informative illustrations which follow. Most specialists in diabetes have seen real-life examples of the disease processes presented in this book but some may be very unfamiliar to the generalist.

For specialists, however, many years of practice are required to accumulate this experience. How often does a non-specialist see a patient with Prader–Willi syndrome, acromegaly or Rabson–Mendenhall syndrome? A quick glance at Figures 9, 12 and 18 will help to imprint the appearances of each of these syndromes. Many physicians caring for people with type 1 DM know of autoimmune destruction of the β-cell, but what exactly does this mean? Figures 27–35 and their legends take the reader through this topic. What is the best way to treat patients with type 1 DM? An important step is to attempt to reproduce the normal fasting and post-prandial insulin profiles. How is this done and what insulin preparations are available to achieve it? Figures 50–62 provide a step-by-step overview aimed at helping the practitioner learn, rather than simply memorize, the requisite information.

Every patient with diabetes should undergo examination of the fundus at least once a year by a physician who is familiar with the manifestations of diabetic retinopathy. This is not always an easy task. How does one distinguish early background retinopathy from the more serious high-risk retinopathy? Figures 81–102, to a large extent, constitute a user's guide to examination of the diabetic fundus. Similarly, Figures 104–34 show excellent examples of other common and not-so-common manifestations of diabetic microvascular and macrovascular complications. A wide array of skin and other manifestations and associations of diabetes is demonstrated.

Many excellent and comprehensive textbooks of diabetes are available, but I am unaware of any other illustrated text with the scope and breadth of Dr Scobie's *Atlas of Diabetes Mellitus*. I am delighted to write a foreword to the third edition of this wonderful and successful Atlas and more than delighted to keep my own personal copy. I have no doubt that both my students and I will continue to find this book useful for many years to come. I suspect that those of you who choose to add this excellent Atlas to your library will find that you will also share my enthusiasm for this delightful book.

Robert A Rizza, MD
Rochester, MN

Preface

The world is witnessing an increase in new cases of diabetes, in both the developed and the developing nations, of near epidemic proportion. This ubiquitous condition will have an ever-increasing impact on all aspects of medicine and public health. It follows that all practicing physicians must seek to gain at least a basic knowledge and understanding of this important global health problem that is so closely linked to the increasing prevalence of obesity.

Diabetes is the paradigm of a condition that necessitates a multidisciplinary approach to its management and treatment. Primary care physicians, hospital physicians, surgeons, nurses, dieticians, psychologists, podiatrists and ophthalmologists are all drawn into this process. In addition, medical students and postgraduate doctors need to learn about diabetes and its protean manifestations.

The third edition of this book continues to build on the previous two editions in providing a clinical and scientific background to the diagnosis, clinical presentations and treatment of diabetes mellitus with a further aim of portraying the wide and varied expressions of diabetes and its complications as an aid to their more ready recognition in clinical practice. It also aims to illustrate the breathtaking developments that are taking place in the field of new therapies for diabetes. This Atlas should, therefore, be of interest to all those who are involved in the provision of diabetic health care and should provide some insight into the fruits of the explosion of basic science and clinical research that has been conducted in an attempt to further our understanding of diabetes and to care better for our diabetic patients.

Ian N Scobie MD FRCP
Gillingham, Kent

Acknowledgments

I wish to extend great thanks to Professor Peter Sönksen and Dr Clara Lowy formerly of St Thomas' Hospital, London, UK, who kindly supplied many of the slides in this Atlas. I am greatly indebted to Dr Tom Barrie, of The Glasgow Eye Infirmary, Glasgow, UK, who provided a splendid set of eye slides (Figures 82, 87, 97 and 99–101), Dr Alan Foulis, of The Royal Infirmary in Glasgow, UK, who supplied some magnificent pathology slides (Figures 23–26, 29–33, 35–39, 41) and Eli Lilly and Company for providing Figures 1–3, 46–49, 51, 54 and 56–60.

I am grateful to the following who also contributed their slides:

Dr Nick Finer, Luton and Dunstable Hospital, Bedfordshire, UK (Figure 8); Professor Ian Campbell, Victoria Hospital, Kirkaldy, Fife, UK (Figures 14 and 106); Dr Sam Chong, Medway Maritime Hospital, Gillingham, Kent, UK (Figure 17); Drs Angus MacCuish and John Quin, formerly The Royal Infirmary, Glasgow, UK (Figure 18); Dr Julian Shield, University of Bristol, UK (Figure 19); Professor Julia Polak, Royal Postgraduate Medical School, Hammersmith, London, UK (Figures 27 and 28); Professor GianFranco Bottazzo, previously The London Hospital Medical College, London, UK (Figure 34); Dr Gray Smith-Laing (Figures 42, 43 and 45) and Dr Richard Day, formerly of Medway Maritime Hospital, Gillingham, Kent, UK (Figure 44); Novo Nordisk Pharmaceuticals Limited, Crawley, UK (Figures 52, 53 and 55); MiniMed, Ashtead, UK (Figures 62 and 69); MediSense, Maidenhead, UK (Figure 67); CDX Diagnostics, Sunderland, Tyne and Wear, UK (Figure 68); Dr David Kerr, Royal Bournemouth Hospital, Dorset, UK (Figures 65, 70–72); Dr William Campbell, Royal Victorian Eye & Ear Hospital, Melbourne, Australia (Figures 90–92); Professor Stephanie Amiel, King's College Hospital, London, UK (Figures 77, 152 and 153); Professor Peter Thomas, Royal Free School of Medicine, Hampstead, London, UK (Figure 104); Mr Grant Fullarton, Gartnavel General Hospital, Glasgow, UK (Figure 110); Pfizer Limited, Sandwich, UK (Figures 111–114, 154); Dr Roger Lindley (Figure 115); Dr Brian Ayres, St Thomas' Hospital, London, UK (Figures 120 and 121); Dr Kumar Segaran, Medway Maritime Hospital, Gillingham, Kent, UK (Figures 122 and 123); Mrs Ali Foster, King's College Hospital, London, UK (Figure 124); Mr Mike Green (Figures 125 and 126), Dr Kishore Reddy (Figure 131), Dr Paul Ryan (Figures 133 and 134), Dr Larry Shall (Figures 136, 140–142, 144) all of Medway Maritime Hospital, Gillingham, Kent, UK; Dr Peter Watkins, King's College Hospital, London, UK (Figure 149); Mr Harry Belcher, Queen Victoria Hospital, East Grinstead, Sussex, UK (Figure 150).

Finally, I thank Mrs Daniella James for typing the text and Mrs Carol Esson and Mrs Elizabeth Cannell for help with previous editions.

Ian N Scobie MD FRCP
Gillingham, Kent

1 Introduction

Diabetes mellitus (DM) is set to become one of the world's biggest health problems owing to the projected increase in new cases.

The word *diabetes* means 'to run through' or 'a siphon' in Greek and the condition has been recognized since the time of the ancient Egyptians. *Mellitus* (from the Latin and Greek roots for 'honey') was later added to the name of this disorder when it became appreciated that diabetic urine tasted sweet.

The incidence of type 1 diabetes differs enormously between populations (in England and Wales the incidence rate is between 15 and 19 cases per 100 000 population per year). There seems to be a slightly higher risk for boys than for girls, at least in high-risk populations. There are peaks of incidence before school age and around puberty with the diagnosis being made more frequently in winter months. An epidemic of type 2 DM is occurring throughout the world, particularly affecting developing countries and migrants from these countries to industrialized societies. Highest prevalence rates are found in some native American tribes, notably the Pima Indians in Arizona (over 50%) and South Pacific groups. Age-standardized prevalence in the UK is 1–2% for the white population, 11% for those of Indian origin and 9% for those of African-Caribbean origin. Rates for the USA are 12–20% for migrant Hispanic groups, 9% for male black African-Americans, 13% for female black African-Americans and 3–8% for non-Hispanic white Americans.

The personal and public health costs of diabetes are high. It has been estimated that diabetes accounts for 2.8% of all hospital admissions in some countries.

The cost of diabetes to society in a developed country may be up to 4.5% of the total health-care costs.

DEFINITION OF DIABETES

DM is a group of metabolic disorders characterized by hyperglycemia. The hyperglycemia results from defects in insulin secretion, insulin action or both. The chronic hyperglycemia of diabetes is associated with specific chronic complications resulting in damage to or failure of various organs, notably the eyes, kidneys, nerves, heart and blood vessels.

DIAGNOSIS OF DIABETES

The diagnostic criteria for DM have been modified in recent years by the American Diabetes Association (ADA) from previous recommendations made by the National Diabetes Data Group in 1979 and the World Health Organization (WHO) in 1985. In clinical practice, establishing the diagnosis of diabetes is seldom a problem. When symptoms of hyperglycemia exist (thirst, polyuria, weight loss, etc.) a random plasma glucose concentration of ≥ 11.1 mmol/l (200 mg/dl) or a fasting plasma glucose (FPG) of ≥ 7.0 mmol/l (126 mg/dl) confirms the diagnosis. Where diagnostic difficulty exists, the precise diagnosis can be established with an oral glucose tolerance test (OGTT) using a 75 g anhydrous glucose load dissolved in water: a 2 h value ≥ 11.1 mmol/l (200 mg/dl) establishes the diagnosis of diabetes. A confirmatory test using one or other of the three methods should be employed. The OGTT is not recommended for routine clinical use, but may be an important test for epidemiologic purposes where using the FPG only may lead to lower prevalence rates than with the combined use of the FPG and OGTT. The ADA recognizes an intermediate group of subjects whose FPG is ≥6.1 mmol/l (110 mg/dl) but <7.0 mmol/l (126 mg/dl) and has defined this group as having impaired fasting glucose (IFG). It has recently been suggested by the ADA that the FPG level to diagnose IFG should be reduced from ≥6.1 mmol/l (110 mg/dl) to ≥5.6 mmol/l (100 mg/dl). A further abnormal category is defined as having a plasma glucose ≥7.8 mmol/l (140 mg/dl) but <11.1 mmol/l (200 mg/dl) at 2 h when an OGTT is used and is described as impaired glucose tolerance (IGT).

CLASSIFICATION OF DIABETES

The diagnostic label 'diabetes mellitus' refers not to a unique disease but rather to multiple disorders of different causation. Increasing knowledge has allowed us to identify discrete conditions caused by specific genetic abnormalities, while other types of diabetes remain difficult to classify on an etiologic basis. The ADA has published a new etiologic classification of diabetes, an adapted version of which is presented in Figure 6.

Type 1 diabetes (previously insulin-dependent diabetes mellitus (IDDM)) is characterized by β-cell destruction, usually leading to absolute insulin deficiency and associated with a usually juvenile onset, a tendency to ketosis and diabetic ketoacidosis, and an absolute need for insulin treatment. Most patients have type 1A diabetes, which is caused by a cellular-mediated autoimmune destruction of the β-cells of the pancreas, a minority have type 1B diabetes the precise etiology of which is not known.

Type 2 diabetes (previously non-insulin-dependent diabetes mellitus (NIDDM)) is associated with obesity and an onset later in life (although cases in childhood are now being recognized in the USA). Patients, at least initially and often throughout their lives, do not have a need for insulin therapy. The disorder manifests as a result of insulin resistance and relative insulin deficiency. A precise cause (or causes) has not been found. This type of diabetes frequently remains undiagnosed for many years despite affected individuals being at risk of developing serious macrovascular or microvascular complications of the disease. Some patients may masquerade as type 2 diabetic patients, but ultimately are recognized as having a late-onset slowly progressing immune-mediated type 1 diabetes, so called latent autoimmune diabetes in adults (LADA).

Specific monogenetic defects of the β-cell have been identified and usually give rise to maturity-onset diabetes of the young (MODY). MODY is defined as a genetic defect in β-cell function subclassified according to the specific gene involved and is described in detail in Chapter 2 in the section 'Other types of diabetes'.

Diabetes may result from any process that adversely affects the pancreas and such acquired processes include pancreatitis, trauma, pancreatectomy and pancreatic cancer. Usually extensive pancreatic damage or removal must occur for diabetes to emerge. Cystic fibrosis, hemochromatosis and fibrocalculous pancreatopathy may also cause diabetes. Diabetes may also be caused by other endocrine diseases particularly when there is over-secretion of hormones that antagonize the normal effect of insulin (including Cushing's syndrome, acromegaly, pheochromocytoma). Drugs that have a similar effect (glucocorticoids, diazoxide, thiazides) may also cause diabetes. Diabetes may also occur as a result of certain rare disorders associated with abnormalities of insulin or the insulin receptor, causing extreme insulin resistance and sometimes found in association with acanthosis nigricans. These disorders are categorized as insulin resistance syndromes. There is a wide array of other genetic syndromes sometimes associated with diabetes, e.g. Down's, Klinefelter's, Turner's syndromes.

Gestational diabetes mellitus (GDM) is defined as any degree of glucose intolerance with onset or first recognition during pregnancy. Care must be taken to exclude type 2 diabetes that was present before pregnancy and type 1 diabetes diagnosed during pregnancy. The patient's glucose tolerance status needs to be re-classified 6 weeks after giving birth. Deterioration of glucose tolerance occurs during normal pregnancy, especially in the third trimester. The criteria for diagnosing abnormal glucose tolerance in pregnancy have not been agreed worldwide: in the USA the modified O'Sullivan–Mahan criteria have been adopted, but these are at variance with the WHO criteria.

Patients with GDM are at future risk of developing type 2 diabetes.

IFG and IGT refer to a pathophysiologic state between normality and frank diabetes. Patients with IGT may only manifest as hyperglycemic when challenged with an oral glucose load. Between 10 and 15% of IGT patients will develop type 2 diabetes within 5 years, although some may return to normal glucose tolerance. Although patients with IGT do not normally develop the microvascular complications of diabetes, they commonly display other features of the insulin resistance syndrome (also known as syndrome X, the metabolic syndrome or Reaven's syndrome), e.g. hypertension and dyslipidemia, and IGT is associated with a major increase in cardiovascular risk.

EPIDEMIOLOGY OF DIABETES

The epidemiology of type 1 diabetes, a disease of as yet unknown etiology, is complex. The overall incidence rates are comparable in North America and Europe; however, this disguises some marked variations in incidence rates between countries and even within countries. Within Europe, particularly high incidence rates are found in Finland, Sweden and Sardinia. Most Asian populations have a low incidence rate. In general, the incidence of type 1 diabetes seems to be increasing with an average increase in incidence of around 3% per year. About half of all cases of type 1 diabetes are diagnosed at an age of < 15 years, with an observed peak in incidence rates in children aged 10–14 years. More recently, many cases are being diagnosed in children of < 5 years of age. In many high-risk populations a male excess of type 1 diabetes is seen, especially after the age of puberty.

Cases of type 2 diabetes greatly exceed those of type 1 diabetes accounting for about 85% of cases in Europe and significantly more than this in certain ethnic groups. It is predicted that the total number of people with diabetes will rise to 300 million, or maybe more, by 2025 with a preponderance of cases occurring in the developing world. In many populations there is a declining age of peak incidence with cases now being identified in children and young adolescents, especially in highly susceptible groups such as Native Americans. In North America, type 2 diabetes is highly prevalent in Native American communities such as the Pima Indians, a feature shared by the Nauru and Papua New Guinea populations of the Pacific Islands. US Hispanic, black Americans and Polynesians also exhibit high prevalence rates. In the UK, prevalence rates of 3–5% are frequently found with higher rates observed in the Asian population as reported also in the Asian subcontinent.

BIBLIOGRAPHY

Alberti KGGM. Preventing insulin dependent diabetes mellitus. Promising strategies but formidable hurdles still to clear. Br Med J 1993; 307: 1435–6

Alberti KG, Zimmet PZ. Definition, diagnosis and classification of diabetes mellitus and its complications. Part I: diagnosis and classification of diabetes mellitus provisional report of a WHO consultation. Diabet Med 1998; 15: 539–53

American Diabetes Association. Type 2 diabetes in children and adolescents. Diabetes Care 2000; 23: 381–9

Diabetes care and research in Europe: the Saint Vincent declaration. Diabet Med 1990; 7: 360

Eisenbarth GS. Type I diabetes mellitus. A chronic autoimmune disease. N Engl J Med 1986; 314: 1360–8

Larsson H, Berglund G, Lindgarde F, Ahren B. Comparison of ADA and WHO criteria for diagnosis of diabetes and glucose intolerance. Diabetologia 1998; 41: 1124–5

MacFarlane IA. Diabetes mellitus and endocrine disease. In Pickup J, Williams G, eds. Textbook of Diabetes. Oxford: Blackwell Scientific Publications, 1991: 263–75

Report of the Expert Committee on the Diagnosis and Classification of Diabetes Mellitus. Diabetes Care 1998; 21 (Suppl): s5–19

Zimmet PZ, Tuomi T, Mackay IR, et al. Latent autoimmune diabetes mellitus in adults (LADA): the role of antibodies to glutamic acid decarboxylase in diagnosis and prediction of insulin dependency. Diabet Med 1994; 11: 299–303

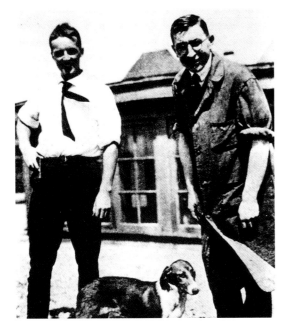

Figure 1 The discovery of insulin in 1922 is accredited to Frederick Banting and Charles Best (a medical student), seen above, supervised by JJR MacLeod and assisted by James Collip. The work was carried out at the University of Toronto

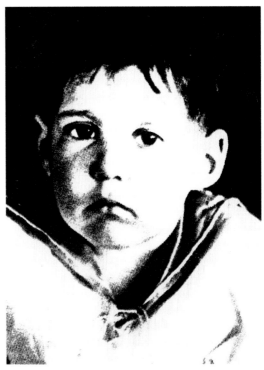

Figure 2 The same child as seen in Figure 2 in 1923 after insulin treatment became available following its discovery by the Toronto group. The effect of this new therapy was 'miraculous'

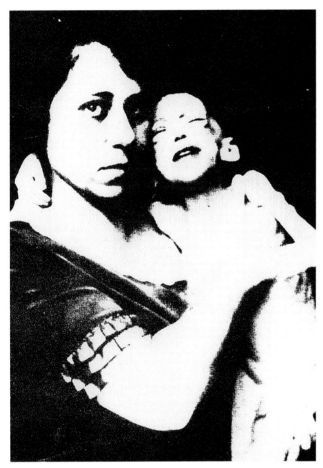

Figure 3 A 3-year-old child with type 1 diabetes mellitus, photographed in 1922 before insulin treatment was available. The only treatment then was a 'starvation' diet; patients rarely survived for more than 2 years

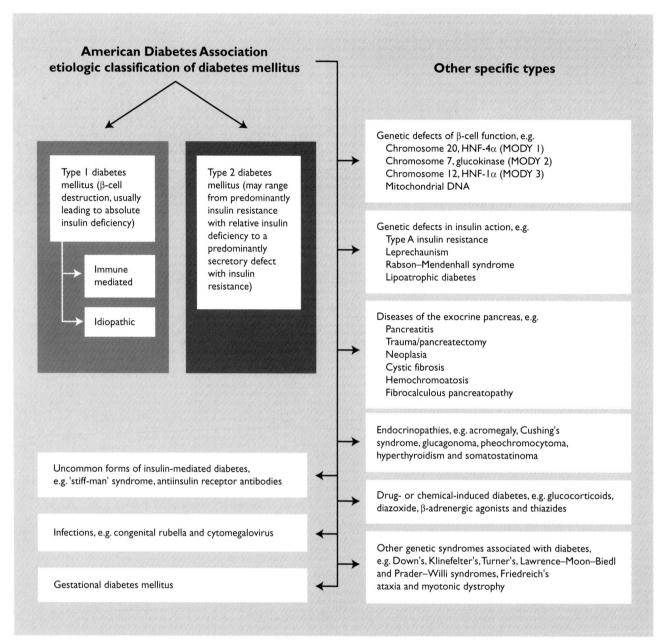

Figure 6 The American Diabetes Association has proposed an etiologic classification of diabetes based on research findings over the past two decades. The nomenclature has changed from insulin-dependent diabetes to type 1 diabetes and from non-insulin diabetes mellitus to type 2 diabetes. All forms of diabetes are characterized according to their known etiologies, immunologic, genetic or otherwise. This opens up the concept of 'the diabetic syndrome'. HNF, hepatic nuclear factor; MODY, maturity-onset diabetes of the young

Diagnosis of diabetes mellitus positive if:

Symptoms of diabetes plus random plasma glucose concentration of ≥ 11.1 mmol/l

or

Fasting plasma glucose concentration of ≥ 7.0 mmol/l

or

Plasma glucose concentration at 2 h ≥ 11.1 mmol/l during a 75 g oral glucose tolerance test
(in the absence of unequivocal hyperglycemia or symptoms, the diagnosis should be
confirmed by repeat testing on a different day)

Figure 7 Although a definitive diagnosis of diabetes may be made using the glucose tolerance test, it is no longer recommended for routine clinical use. In the presence of diabetic symptoms, the diagnosis may be established by finding a random plasma glucose level of ≥ 11.1 mmol/l (200 mg/dl) or a fasting plasma glucose level of ≥ 7.0 mmol/l (126 mg/dl). Both impaired fasting glucose and impaired glucose tolerance are defined in the text

2 Pathogenesis

TYPE I DIABETES MELLITUS

Type 1 diabetes mellitus (DM) is a disease of multi-factorial autoimmune causation. Worldwide, there is a marked geographic variation in prevalence. The overall lifetime risk in Caucasian subjects is approximately 0–4%. Type 1 DM is caused by an interaction between environmental factors and an inherited genetic predisposition. In twin studies, a significant genetic contribution is suggested by a concordance value for type 1 DM of 30–50%. The risk to a first-degree relative is approximately 5%. The high discordance rate supports the notion that type 1 DM is multifactorial in etiology. Environmental triggers may account for up to two-thirds of the disease susceptibility.

About 20 different regions of the human genome have been found to have some degree of linkage with type 1 DM. To date, the strongest linkage has been with genes encoded in the human leukocyte antigen (HLA) region located within the major histocompatibility complex (MHC), the contribution of which to disease risk is now designated IDDM1. This appears to be the most powerful determinant of genetic susceptibility to the disease, accounting for approximately 40% of familial inheritance. More than 90% of patients who develop type 1 DM have either DR3, DQ2 or DR4, DQγ haplotypes, whereas fewer than 40% of normal controls have these haplotypes. DR3-DR4 heterozygosity is highest in children who develop diabetes before the age of 5 years (50%) and lowest in adults presenting with type 1 diabetes (20–30%) compared with an overall US population prevalence of 2.4%. Specific polymorphisms of the DQB1 gene

encoding the β-chain of class II DQ molecules predispose to diabetes in Caucasians but not in Japanese. In contrast, the HLS-DQ6 molecule protects against the disease. HLA antigens (classes I and II) are cell-surface glycoproteins that play a crucial role in presenting autoantigen peptide fragments to T lymphocytes and thus initiating an immune response. Polymorphisms in the genes encoding specific peptide chains of the HLA molecules may therefore modulate the ability of β-cell-derived antigens to trigger an autoimmune response against the β-cell.

Only one non-HLA gene has been identified with certainty and that is the insulin gene (INS) region on chromosome 11p5.5, now designated IDDM2. Population studies of Caucasian type 1 diabetic subjects and non-diabetic controls initially showed a positive association between alleles within the INS region and disease susceptibility. However, recent genome screens have provided conflicting data regarding the role of the INS gene region (IDDM2). It is thought that INS and HLA act independently in the causation of type 1 diabetes and that the INS gene region (IDDM2) accounts for 10% of familial clustering.

The most likely environmental factor implicated in the causation of type 1 DM is viral infection. Numerous viruses attack the pancreatic β-cell either directly through a cytolytic effect or by triggering an autoimmune attack against the β-cell. Evidence for a viral factor in etiology has come from animal models and, in humans, from observation of seasonal and geographic variations in the onset of the disease. In addition, patients newly presenting with type 1 DM may exhibit serologic evidence of viral infection. Viruses that have been linked to human type 1 DM include mumps, Coxsackie B, retroviruses, rubella, cytomegalovirus and Epstein–Barr virus. Bovine serum albumin, a major constituent of cow's milk, has been implicated as a cause of type 1 DM in children exposed at an early age, but definitive proof is lacking and this remains controversial. Nitrosamines (found in smoked and cured meats) may be diabetogenic as may chemicals known to be toxic to pancreatic β-cells, including alloxan, streptozotocin and the rat poison Vacor. Recent reports suggesting that early ingestion of cereal or gluten increases the risk of type 1 diabetes remain to be confirmed.

Type 1 DM is associated with autoimmune destruction of the β-cells of the endocrine pancreas. Examination of islet tissue obtained from pancreatic biopsy or at postmortem from patients with recent-onset type 1 DM confirms a mononuclear cell infiltrate (termed insulitis) with the presence of CD4 and CD8 T lymphocytes, B lymphocytes and macrophages suggesting that these cells have a role in the destruction of β-cells. Although the precise mechanism of such an insult has not been elucidated it seems likely that an environmental factor, such as a viral infection, in a subject with an inherited predisposition to the disease, triggers the damaging immune response. This results in aberrant expression of class II MHC antigen by pancreatic β-cells. T lymphocytes recognize antigen-presenting cells and are activated, producing cytokines such as interleukin (IL)-2, interferon (IFN)γ and tumor necrosis factor (TNF)-α. This generates a clone of T lymphocytes that carry receptors specific to the presented antigen. Such T-helper cells assist B lymphocytes to produce antibodies directed against the β-cell. Such antibodies include islet cell antibodies (ICA) directed against cytoplasmic components of the islet cells. ICA presence may precede the development of type 1 DM. Some subjects may develop ICA temporarily and not go on to develop the disease, but persistence of ICA leads to progressive β-cell destruction associated with the chronic inflammatory cell infiltrate termed 'insulitis'. Type 1 DM ensues. Other antibodies associated with type 1 DM are islet cell-surface antibodies (present in 30–60% of newly diagnosed type 1 DM patients), insulin autoantibodies (IAA) and antibodies to an isoform of glutamic acid decarboxylase (GAD).

TYPE 2 DIABETES MELLITUS

Type 2 DM is one of the most commonly seen genetic disorders, yet its exact mode of inheritance has remained elusive and is likely to be polygenic. The rate of concordance is high in identical twins, but is much lower in non-identical dizygotic twins. Patients with type 2 DM show an increased frequency of diabetes in other family members compared with the non-diabetic population. Only a small proportion of patients (< 3%) with type 2 DM have a monogenic disorder. No unequivocal, reproducible associations with type 2 diabetes have been found for candidate genes studied so far. Furthermore, no genome scans in type 2 DM have identified any region with an effect as large as the HLA region in type 1 DM.

It has long been recognized that the hyperglycemia of type 2 DM results from a defect in both insulin secretion and insulin action

Pathogenesis of type 2 DM

Subjects with type 2 DM exhibit abnormalities in glucose homeostasis owing to impaired insulin secretion, insulin resistance in muscle, liver and adipocytes and abnormalities of splanchnic glucose uptake.

Insulin secretion in type 2 DM

Impaired insulin secretion is a universal finding in patients with type 2 diabetes. In the early stages of type 2 DM insulin resistance can be compensated for by an increase in insulin secretion leading to normal glucose tolerance. With increasing insulin resistance, the fasting plasma glucose will rise, accompanied by an increase in fasting plasma insulin levels, until a fasting plasma glucose level is reached when the β-cell is unable to maintain its elevated rate of insulin secretion at which point the fasting plasma insulin declines sharply. Hepatic glucose production will begin to rise. When fasting plasma glucose reaches high levels, the plasma insulin response to a glucose challenge is markedly blunted. Although fasting insulin levels remain elevated, postprandial insulin and C-peptide secretory rates are decreased. This natural history of type 2 diabetes starting from normal glucose tolerance, followed by insulin resistance, compensatory hyperinsulinemia and then by progression to impaired glucose tolerance and overt diabetes has been documented in a variety of populations.

Type 2 DM is characterized by loss of the first-phase insulin response to an intravenous glucose load, although this abnormality may be acquired secondary to glucotoxicity. Loss of the first-phase insulin response is important as this early quick insulin secretion primes insulin target tissues, especially the liver.

There may be multiple possible causes of the impaired insulin secretion in type 2 DM with several abnormalities having been shown to disturb the delicate balance between islet neogenesis and apoptosis. Studies in first-degree relatives of patients with type 2 diabetes and in twins have provided strong evidence for the genetic basis of abnormal β-cell function. Acquired defects in type 2 diabetes may lead to impairment of insulin secretion. Clinical studies in man, and animal studies, have supported the concept of glucotoxicity, whereby an elevation in plasma glucose levels, in the presence of a reduced β-cell mass, can lead to a major impairment in insulin secretion. Lipotoxicity has also been implicated as an acquired cause of impaired β-cell function. Patients with type 2 DM exhibit a reduced response of the incretin glucagon-like peptide (GLP)-1 in response to oral glucose, while GLP-1 administration enhances the postprandial insulin secretory response and may restore near-normal glycemia.

Amyloid deposits (islet amyloid polypeptide (IAPP)) or amylin in the pancreas are frequently observed in patients with type 2 diabetes and have been implicated as a cause of progressive β-cell failure. However, definitive evidence that amylin contributes to β-cell dysfunction in humans is lacking.

Insulin resistance in type 2 DM

Insulin resistance is a characteristic feature of both lean and obese individuals with type 2 diabetes. As indicated above, in the fasting state, plasma insulin levels are increased in patients with type 2 diabetes. Since hyperinsulinemia is a potent inhibitor of hepatic glucose production and an excessive rate of hepatic glucose production is the major abnormality responsible for the elevated fasting plasma glucose in type 2 diabetes, it follows that there must be hepatic resistance to the action of insulin. The liver is also resistant to the inhibitory effect of hyperglycemia on hepatic

glucose output. Most of the increase in hepatic glucose production can be accounted for by an increase in hepatic gluconeogenesis.

Muscle is the major site of insulin-stimulated glucose disposal in humans. Muscle represents the primary site of insulin resistance in type 2 diabetic subjects leading to a marked blunting of glucose uptake into peripheral muscle. In contrast, splanchnic tissues, like the brain, are relatively insensitive to insulin with respect to stimulation of glucose uptake. Following glucose ingestion both impaired suppression of hepatic glucose production and decreased muscle glucose uptake are responsible for the observed glucose intolerance leading to hyperglycemia.

There is a dynamic relationship between insulin resistance and impaired insulin secretion. Insulin resistance is an early and characteristic feature of type 2 diabetes in high-risk populations. Overt diabetes develops only when the β-cells are unable to increase sufficiently their insulin output to compensate for the defect in insulin action (insulin resistance).

Insulin resistance in type 2 diabetes is primarily due to post-binding defects in insulin action. Diminished insulin binding is modest and secondary to down-regulation of the insulin receptor by chronic hyperglycemia. Post-binding defects that have been recognized include reduced insulin receptor tyrosine kinase activity, insulin signal transduction abnormalities, decreased glucose transport, diminished glucose phosphorylation and impaired glycogen synthase activity. Quantitatively, impaired glycogen synthesis represents the major abnormality responsible for insulin resistance in type 2 diabetic patients.

OTHER TYPES OF DIABETES

Maturity-onset diabetes of the young (MODY) is inherited as an autosomal dominant and, to date, abnormalities at six genetic loci on different chromosomes have been identified. The most common form of MODY is associated with mutations on chromosome 12 in hepatic nuclear factor (HNF)-1α and hence this is referred to as transcription-factor MODY. Other mutations affect such transcription factors as HNF-1β, HNF-4α, insulin promoter factor-1 and NEUROD 1. Transcription factor mutations alter insulin secretion in the mature β-cell as well as altering β-cell development, proliferation and cell death.

Glucose tolerance is normal at birth, but progressive β-cell dysfunction ensues until the emergence of frank diabetes. Patients with transcription-factor mutations tend to be lean and insulin-sensitive rather than obese and insulin-resistant. Microvascular complications are frequent.

The first gene implicated in MODY was the glucokinase gene. Mutations on the glucokinase gene on chromosome 7p result in a defective glucokinase molecule. As glucokinase converts glucose to glucose-6-phosphate, the metabolism of which stimulates insulin secretion by the β-cell, glucokinase serves as a 'glucose sensor'. With defects in the glucokinase gene, increased plasma levels of glucose are necessary to elicit normal levels of insulin secretion. Over 100 glucokinase gene mutations have now been found in families from several different countries. Fasting hyperglycemia is present from birth and worsens very slowly with age. Subjects are usually detected by screening, e.g. in pregnancy or during coincidental illness or by family studies. The mild hyperglycemia of this type of MODY rarely needs any treatment other than diet, and microvascular complications are rare.

Other specific genetic defects leading to diabetes include point mutations in mitochondrial DNA, genetic abnormalities leading to the inability to convert proinsulin to insulin and to the production of mutant insulin molecules and mutations of the insulin receptor.

As previously described, diabetes may result from overt diseases of the exocrine pancreas, secondary to specific endocrinopathies and due to drugs or chemicals. Certain viruses have been associated with β-cell destruction (Coxsackievirus B, cytomegalovirus, adenovirus, mumps, congenital rubella), although in most cases the precise nature of the association remains unclear. Many other genetic syndromes are accompanied by an increased incidence of diabetes (Down's syndrome, Klinefelter's syndrome, Turner's syndrome, Wolfram's syndrome).

THE OBESITY EPIDEMIC

A dramatic increase in the prevalence of obesity has been witnessed in many countries in the past quarter of a century. Obesity, at least in Caucasian populations, is defined as a body mass index (BMI; weight (kg)/height (m)^2) over 30 (a lower level has been suggested for some ethnic groups.) BMI may not accurately reflect fat mass nor its distribution. Fairly accurate estimations of fat distribution may be gained by measuring the waist–hip ratio or more simply waist circumference, both of which correlate well with more sophisticated techniques, such as computed tomography or magnetic resonance imaging. The measurement of waist circumference has become part of the definition of the metabolic syndrome or syndrome X, a condition that predisposes to the development of type 2 diabetes. Since 1980 the prevalence of obesity in the UK has risen from 6% in men and 8% in women to 19% in men and 21% in women in 1999 and since then it has risen still further. In the USA, the prevalence of obesity has increased between the period 1976–1980 and the period 1999–2000 by 110% such that 65% of the adult population is overweight or obese. Perhaps even more worrying, there has been an alarming increase in weight in children and teenagers in the USA, with more than 10% of 2–5-year olds and 15% of 6–19-year olds being overweight as defined as a BMI ≥95th centile for age and gender. Prevalence rates of obesity have increased more in minority groups as compared with white groups, but people of all ages, races, ethnicities, socioeconomic levels and geographic areas are experiencing a substantial increase in weight. Such data have led to the coining of the term the obesity epidemic, sometimes stated as the obesity pandemic, as this problem is not confined to the developed nations of the world but is also happening in developing nations, particularly in affluent strata of society.

Food intake

It is clear that obesity results from the interaction of many factors including genetic, metabolic, behavioral and environmental influences, but the rapidity with which obesity is increasing, in the context of a relatively stable gene pool, suggests that environmental and behavioral factors largely explain the epidemic. National trends in food consumption have revealed conflicting data; however, ecologic data seem to support the notion that energy intake has increased perhaps related to an increased percentage of food consumed outside the home including fast foods, greater consumption of soft drinks and larger portion sizes.

Energy expenditure

Although it is difficult to quantify, it seems likely that a major downward change in physical activity, and thus energy expenditure, plays a significant role in the development of obesity in modern society whether or not energy intake has increased. This includes the level of activity required at work and in the home, reduced dependence on walking and cycling for transportation, reduced physical activity in schools and more jobs being of a sedentary nature. Of the US population 60% do not participate in regular physical activity and 25% are almost entirely sedentary. Almost half of young Americans are not vigorously active on a routine basis. A cross-sectional study in South Carolina suggested that obese children spent less time in moderate and vigorous physical activity than their non-obese counterparts, and in a national US study, children who engaged in the least vigorous physical activity or the most television viewing tended to be the most overweight.

Sequelae of obesity

Obesity is associated with an increased risk of heart disease, hypertension, a variety of cancers, cerebrovascular disease, gallstones and osteoarthritis; furthermore it has also been associated with an alarming increase in the prevalence of type 2 diabetes with adults presenting at an ever earlier age and the disturbing appearance of type 2 diabetes in adolescents and even children. The health and economic consequences of this are likely to be devastating, thus the obesity epidemic has to be considered a global issue of major importance. Governments and their politicians must address this issue and develop workable public health policies and legislation to reverse the obesity trend.

PREVENTION OF DIABETES

Type 1 diabetes

The National Institute of Diabetes and Digestive and Kidney Diseases (NIDDK) in the USA has set up the type 1 Diabetes Trial Net, a clinical trials network that will explore new treatments in patients with newly presenting diabetes, in family members at risk of developing type 1 diabetes and, possibly, also in people who are at high genetic risk. At present no such therapy has proven to be effective or clinically safe. On the basis of the theory that immune-mediated type 1 diabetes is believed to result from immunologic destruction of islet β-cells as a consequence of an interplay between genetic susceptibility and a triggering environmental agent or agents, it would seem possible to identify potential targets for prevention of the disease, although we know that the above theory is very much an over-simplification of the true pathological mechanism. The development of type 1 diabetes is a slow process with the best prospect of preventive strategies being early in the disease process. At that stage, disease prediction is less accurate and any treatment would need to be safe and harmless, otherwise individuals may come to harm with treatment who were never going to develop the disease. No such agent yet exists.

Strategies to prevent type 1 diabetes would include (a) identification and elimination of environmental triggers, (b) identification and promotion of environmental protective factors and (c) interruption of the immunologic process leading to β-cell destruction.

Several trials have demonstrated that immunosuppressive agents can slow or interrupt the disease process, but concern remains about long-term toxicity. Studies with newer agents (e.g. sirolimus, mycophenolate, etc.) have been initiated. Early studies with anti-CD3 monoclonal antibodies have suggested a beneficial effect on preservation of β-cell function. Nicotinamide has been suggested as a means of protecting β-cells; however, unfortunately a large scale trial (ENDIT: the European Nicotinamide Diabetes Intervention Trial) showed no significant benefit. Expansion of β-cell mass (with exendin, GLP-1 or islet neogenesis-associated protein) is a possible research consideration. Rest of β-cells (with insulin therapy) in early-onset diabetes or ICA-positive relatives has not yet shown conclusively that it delays or prevents the development of type 1 diabetes. More recently several groups have made progress towards the development of a vaccine to prevent the onset of type 1 diabetes.

Type 2 diabetes

Given the expanding prevalence rates of type 2 diabetes both in developed and developing nations, the prevention of type 2 diabetes assumes global importance. Clearly the prevention of type 2 diabetes is incestuously related to the prevention of obesity. Type

2 diabetes lends itself to potential preventative action because of the long delay between development of the earliest metabolic defects and full expression of the disease. Lifestyle modification or pharmacologic intervention that can improve insulin sensitivity (reduce insulin resistance) or improve or preserve β-cell function would expect to have an impact on the future development of type 2 diabetes.

The first major trial to show the effect of lifestyle change on the development of diabetes was the Da Qing Study in China where patients with impaired glucose tolerance (IGT) were randomized to a control group and one of three active treatment groups (change in diet, exercise or change in diet plus exercise). The diet group experienced a relative risk reduction of progression to frank diabetes of 31%, the exercise group of 46% and the combined group of 42%.

This study was followed by the Finnish Diabetes Prevention Study which compared lifestyle intervention to a control group in overweight patients with IGT. The lifestyle intervention group received detailed dietary advice and individualized advice on physical activity with supervized training sessions. During the first year of the study, the intervention group achieved a significant loss of 4.2 kg with minimal change in the control group and after 2 years, the cumulative incidence of progression to diabetes was reduced by 58%. Whether such an intensity of lifestyle intervention could be provided, funded and adhered to outside the context of a clinical trial remains open to debate.

In the USA, the investigators in the Diabetes Prevention Program randomly assigned patients with IGT to one of three arms: placebo, lifestyle modification or metformin (850 mg twice daily). Patients in the lifestyle intervention group were asked to achieve and maintain a reduction of at least 7% in body weight through a healthy diet and to engage in moderate physical activity for at least 150 min per week. Patients received intensive support and, as for the Finnish study, such a level of support is unlikely to be available in routine clinical practice. The lifestyle group achieved a greater weight loss (5.6 kg) and a greater increase in physical activity than the other groups. At 3 years, the prevalence of type 2 diabetes was reduced by 58% with lifestyle change and by 31% in the metformin group.

The multinational STOP-NIDDM Trial (The Study to Prevent Non-Insulin Dependent Diabetes) used acarbose to prevent progression to diabetes in IGT subjects. Patients who were randomized to acarbose were 25% less likely to develop diabetes and when the data were corrected to the revised ADA criteria for the diagnosis of diabetes, there was an even greater relative risk reduction of 32%. Treatment with a glitazone has also been shown to reduce the number of patients who develop diabetes 30 months after gestational diabetes with a 55% relative risk reduction in the TRI-POD study (Troglitazone in Prevention of Diabetes Study).

Several other type 2 diabetes pharmacologic prevention trials are currently being conducted (NAVIGATOR – nateglinide and valsartan, DREAM – ramipril and rosiglitazone, ACT NOW – pioglitazone and ORIGIN – insulin glargine) and their outcome is awaited with interest.

Thus, it has been conclusively shown that lifestyle modification and drug therapy can delay the onset of type 2 diabetes. Whether there has been true 'prevention' in those subjects who did not develop diabetes is a different matter. Cost-effective analyses have not been conducted, although individual health benefit is likely to ensue.

The American Diabetes Association Working Group on the Prevention of Diabetes recommends a lifestyle intervention strategy for patients with IFG (impaired fasting glucose) or IGT but does not recommend routine prescription of drug therapy until more is known about the cost-effectiveness of such a policy.

BIBLIOGRAPHY

Andersen RE, Crespo CJ, Bartlett SJ, et al. Relationship of physical activity and television watching with body weight and level of fatness among children: results from the Third National Health and Nutrition Examination Survey. JAMA 1998; 279: 938–42

Atkinson MA, Eisenbarth GS. Type I diabetes: new perspectives on disease pathogenesis and treatment. Lancet 2001; 358: 221–9

Bottazzo GF. Death of a beta cell: homicide or suicide? Diabetic Med 1986; 3: 119–30

Chiasson JL, Gomis R, Hanefeld M, et al. The STOP-NIDDM Trial: an international study on the efficacy of an alpha-glucosidase inhibitor to prevent type 2 diabetes in a population with impaired glucose tolerance: rationale, design, and preliminary screening data. Study to Prevent Non-Insulin-Dependent Diabetes Mellitus. Diabetes Care 1998; 21: 1720–5

DeFronzo R. The triumvirate: β-cell, muscle, liver. A collusion responsible for NIDDM. Diabetes 1988; 37: 667–75

DeFronzo RA. Pathogenesis of type 2 diabetes mellitus. Med Clin North Am 2004; 88: 787–835

Devendra D, Liu E, Eisenbarth GS. Type 1 diabetes: recent developments. Br Med J 2004; 328: 750–4

Ebbeling CB, Pawiak DB, Ludwig DS. Childhood obesity: public-health crisis, common sense cure. Lancet 2002; 360: 473–82

Froguel P, Velho G. Genetic determinants of type 2 diabetes. Recent Prog Horm Res 2001; 56: 91–105

Fujimoto WY. The importance of insulin resistance in the pathogenesis of type 2 diabetes mellitus. Am J Med 2000; 108 (Suppl 6a): 9s–14s

Hitman GA. The major histocompatibility complex and insulin dependent (type I) diabetes. Autoimmunity 1989; 4: 119–30

Inzucchi SE, Sherwin RS. The prevention of type 2 diabetes mellitus. Endocrinol Metab Clin North Am 2005; 34: 199–219

Kahn SE. The importance of the beta-cell in the pathogenesis of type 2 diabetes mellitus. Am J Med 2000; 108 (Suppl 6a): 2s–8s

Redondo MJ, Fain PR, Eisenbarth GS. Genetics of type IA diabetes. Recent Prog Horm Res 2001; 56: 69–89

Skyler JS. Immunotherapy for interdicting the type 1 diabetes disease process. In Pickup J, Williams G, eds. Textbook of Diabetes, 3rd edn. Oxford: Blackwell Scientific Publications, 2003: 74.1–74.12

Stein CJ, Colditz GA. The epidemic of obesity. J Clin Endocrinol Metab 2004; 89: 2522–5

Szopa TM, Titchener PA, Portwood ND, Taylor KW. Diabetes mellitus due to viruses – some recent developments. Diabetologia 1993; 36: 687–95

Trost SG, Kerr LM, Ward DS, Pate RR. Physical activity and determinates of physical activity in obese and non-obese children. Int J Obes Relat Metab Disord 2001; 25: 822–9

Undlien DE, Lie BA, Thorsby E. HLA complex genes in type I diabetes and other autoimmune diseases. Which genes are involved? Trends Genet 2001; 17: 93–100

Zimmet PZ. The pathogenesis and prevention of diabetes in adults. Genes, autoimmunity, and demography. Diabetes Care 1995; 18: 1050–64

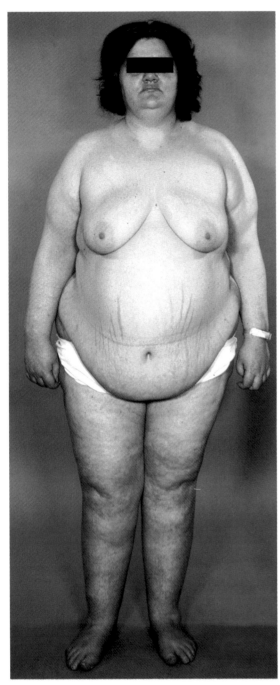

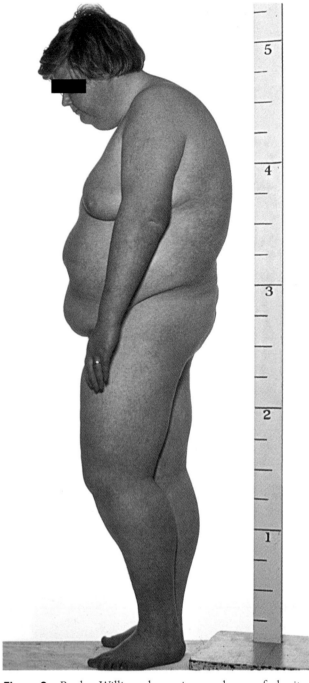

Figure 8 Type 2 diabetes mellitus (DM) is strongly associated with obesity and this link has been recognized for centuries. The risk of developing type 2 DM increases progressively with rising body mass index. Type 2 DM is the result of increased insulin resistance and insulin deficiency. Obesity is strongly associated with insulin resistance and high fasting insulin levels. It has been proposed that this may ultimately result in β-cell failure and the emergence of type 2 DM; however, this theory is oversimplistic and the precise cause of type 2 DM remains unknown except in a few cases of identified genetic abnormalities

Figure 9 Prader–Willi syndrome is a syndrome of obesity, muscular hypotonia, hypogonadotropic hypogonadism and mental retardation associated, in around 50% of cases, with a deletion or translocation of chromosome 15. A small percentage of patients have type 2 diabetes mellitus

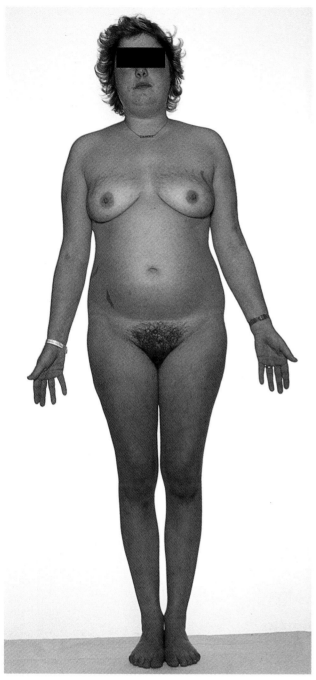

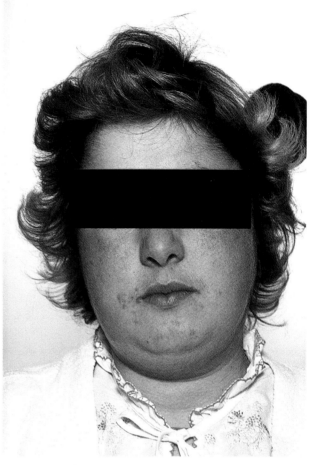

Figure 11 This young woman (same patient as in Figure 10) has the typical facies of Cushing's syndrome – a rounded plethoric face and mild hirsutism. Glucose tolerance is impaired in most patients with Cushing's syndrome and around 25% of patients are diabetic. However, many older patients with type 2 diabetes mellitus have features of Cushing's syndrome, specifically, obesity, hirsutism, hypertension, striae and diabetes, but do not have the condition

Figure 10 The centripetal obesity and prominent lipid striae suggest that this is Cushing's syndrome and not simple obesity

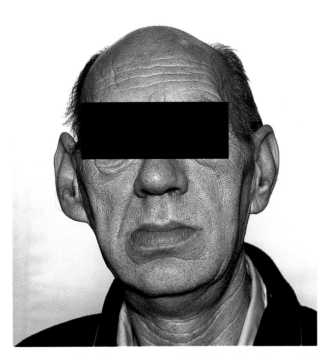

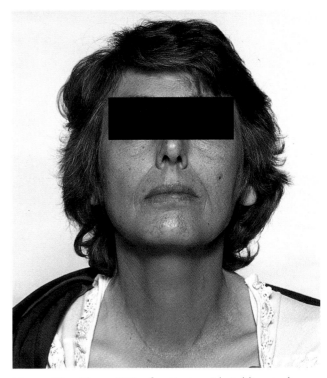

Figure 12 Diabetes occurs in 15–30% of patients with acromegaly and similarly with impaired glucose tolerance. The excess growth hormone secretion, usually from a pituitary adenoma, is associated with insulin resistance which, after several years, may result in the diabetic state. The diabetes is usually type 2, and is associated with the usual microvascular and other complications. Glucose tolerance improves after successful treatment of the acromegaly

Figure 13 About 10% of patients with Addison's disease have diabetes, usually type 1. Diabetic patients who develop Addison's disease exhibit an increased sensitivity to insulin which is reversed by glucocorticoid replacement therapy. Addison's disease and associated type 1 DM or other autoimmune endocrinopathy (such as hypothyroidism, Graves' disease, hypoparathyroidism) is referred to as Schmidt's syndrome

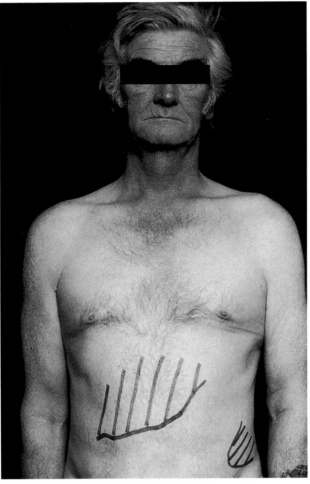

Figure 14 This patient has hereditary hemochromatosis transmitted by an autosomal recessive gene. It occurs most commonly as a result of a mutation in a gene *HFE* – on the short arm of chromosome 6. Patients present with the classic triad of bronze skin pigmentation, hepatomegaly and diabetes mellitus (hence the term 'bronze diabetes'). Cardiac manifestations and pituitary dysfunction also occur

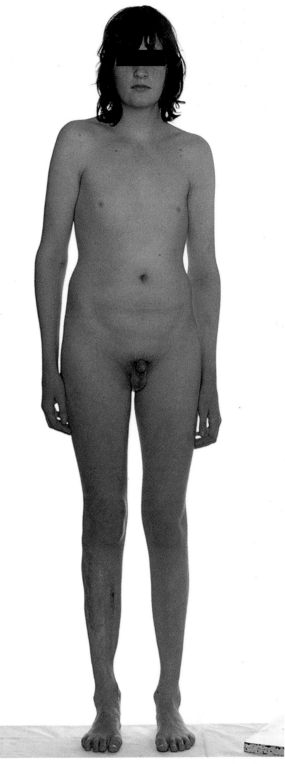

Figure 15 Of the patients who have Klinefelter's syndrome (47,XXY karyotype), 26% show diabetes on the oral glucose tolerance test, but overt symptomatic diabetes is unusual. The cause of the diabetes is not known, but may be related to insulin resistance

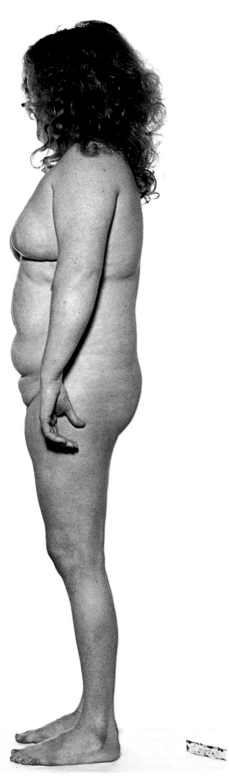

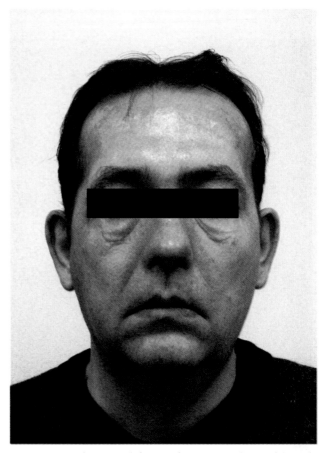

Figure 17 The typical facies of myotonic dystrophy, with frontal balding and a smooth forehead, is associated, albeit rarely, with diabetes mellitus. Impaired glucose tolerance with insulin resistance is more commonly found

Figure 16 Diabetes is present in around 60% of young adults with Turner's syndrome (45,XO karyotype) and is usually type 2. A paradoxic rise in growth hormone to oral glucose may be the cause of the glucose intolerance

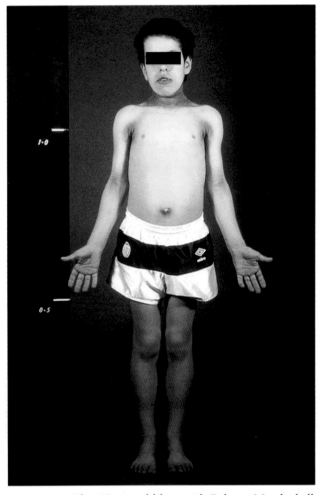

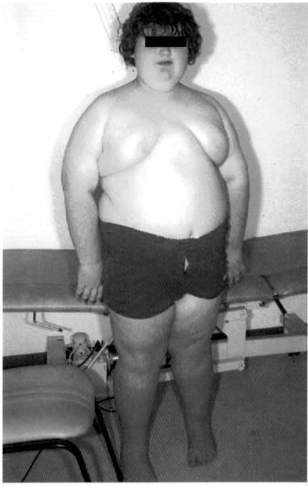

Figure 18 This 13-year-old boy with Rabson–Mendenhall syndrome exhibits severe insulin resistance (moderate hyperglycemia associated with gross elevation of plasma insulin levels). Typically associated features include stunted growth and acanthosis nigricans, affecting the neck, axillae and antecubital fossae, and a characteristic facies

Figure 19 This young child has morbid obesity. As the age of peak incidence of diabetes declines, cases of type 2 diabetes are now being identified in such children and in young adolescents, especially in highly susceptible ethnic groups. The health consequences of this phenomenon are likely to be immense

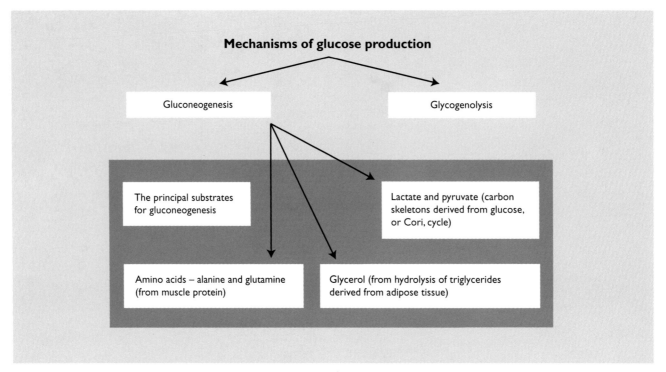

Figure 20 Glucose is produced in the liver by the process of gluconeogenesis and glycogenolysis. The main substrates for gluconeogenesis are the glucogenic amino acids (alanine and glutamine), glycerol, lactate and pyruvate. Many factors influence the rate of gluconeogenesis; it is suppressed by insulin and stimulated by the sympathetic nervous system. Glycogenolysis (the breakdown of hepatic glycogen to release glucose) is stimulated by glucagon and catecholamines, but is inhibited by insulin

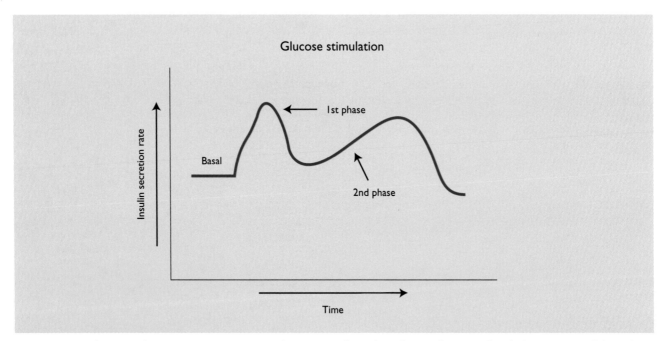

Figure 21 Biphasic insulin response to a constant glucose stimulus: when the β-cell is stimulated, there is a rapid first-phase insulin response 1–3 min after the glucose level is increased; this returns towards baseline 6–10 min later. Thereafter, there is a gradual second-phase insulin response that persists for the duration of the stimulus. Type 2 diabetes mellitus is characterized by loss of the first-phase insulin response and a diminished second-phase response

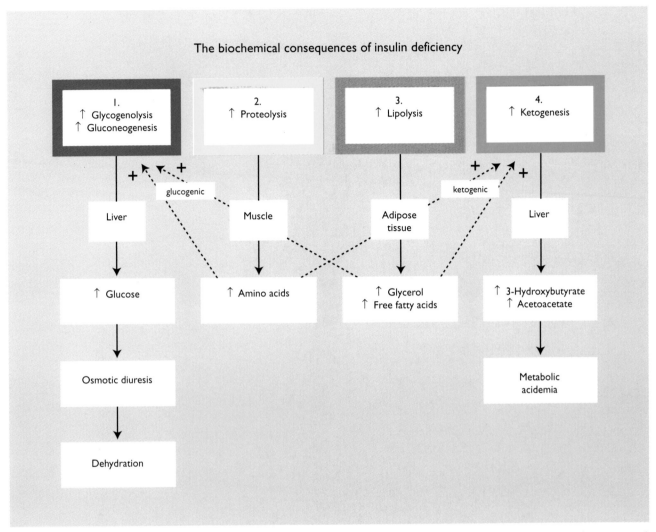

Figure 22 Insulin deficiency results in increased hepatic glucose production and, hence, hyperglycemia by increased gluconeogenesis and glycogenolysis. Insulin deficiency also results in increased proteolysis releasing both glucogenic and ketogenic amino acids. Lipolysis is increased, elevating both glycerol and non-esterified fatty acid levels which further contribute to gluconeogenesis and ketogenesis, respectively. The end result is hyperglycemia, dehydration, breakdown of body fat and protein, and acidemia

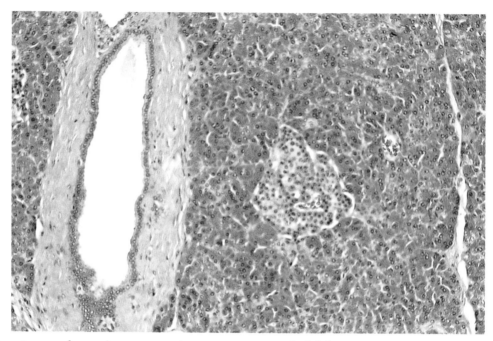

Figure 23 Constituents of normal pancreas, medium-power view: to the left lies an excretory duct and, to the right, there is an islet surrounded by exocrine acinar cells. Hematoxylin and eosin stain

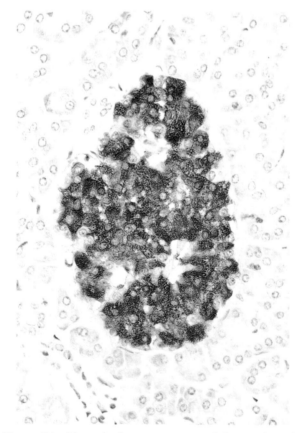

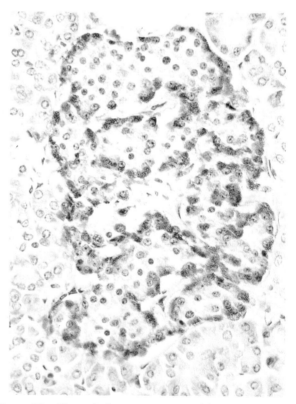

Figure 24 Normal islet immunostained for insulin. The majority (80%) of the endocrine cells are β-cells

Figure 25 Normal islet immunostained for glucagon. Note that the α-cells mark the periphery of blocks of endocrine cells within the islet. Most of the cells within these blocks are β-cells

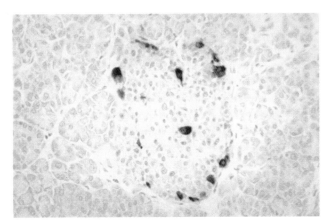

Figure 26 Normal islet immunostained for somatostatin. Somatostatin is contained in the D cells which are scattered within the islet. Somatostatin has an extremely wide range of actions. It inhibits the secretion of insulin, growth hormone and glucagon and also suppresses the release of various gut peptides. Somatostatinomas (D cell tumors) cause weight loss, malabsorption, gallstones, hypochlorhydria and diabetes

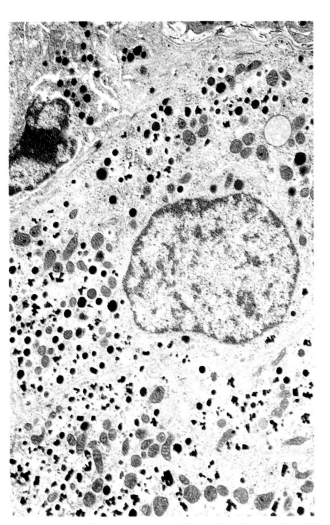

Figure 27 Electron micrograph (EM) of an islet of Langerhans from a normal pancreas showing mainly insulin storage granules in a pancreatic β-cell. A larger α-cell is also seen. The normal adult pancreas contains around 1 million islets comprising mainly β-cells (producing insulin), α-cells (glucagon), D cells (somatostatin) and PP (pancreatic polypeptide) cells. Islet cell types can be distinguished by various histologic stains and by the EM appearances of the secretory granules (as seen here). They can also be identified by immunocytochemical staining of the peptide hormones on light or electron microscopy (see Figures 24 and 25)

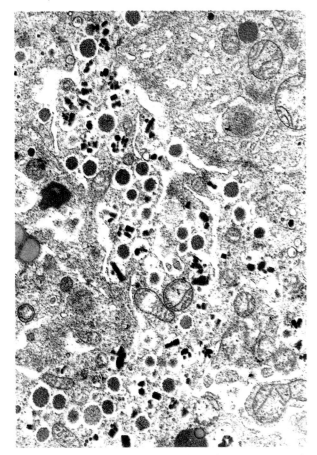

Figure 28 Electron micrograph of insulin storage granules (higher power view than in Figure 27) in a patient with an insulinoma

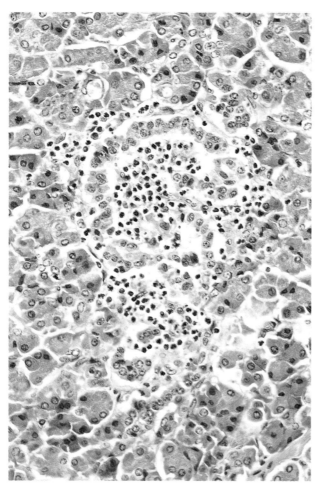

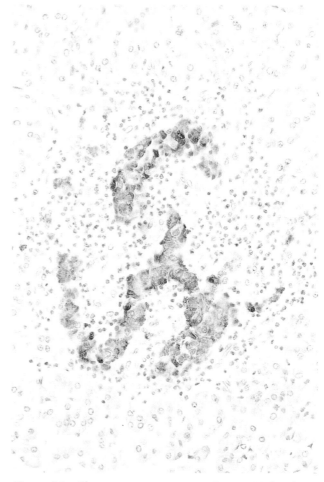

Figure 29 Insulitis. Histologic section of pancreas from a child who died at clinical presentation of type 1 diabetes mellitus. There is a heavy, chronic, inflammatory cell infiltrate affecting the islet. H & E

Figure 30 The same pancreas as in Figure 29 has been immunostained to show β-cells: note the destruction of the β-cells in this islet owing to inflammation; compare with Figure 24

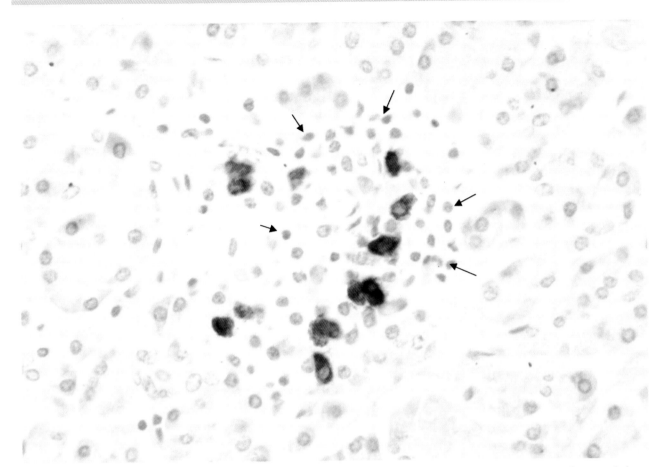

Figure 31 This histologic section of pancreas was obtained at autopsy from a patient 5 years after the onset of type 1 diabetes. It shows persistence of an infiltrate of lymphocytes (insulitis) some of which have been indicated by arrows, affecting this islet, immunostained for insulin. This shows that β-cell destruction takes place over years in patients with type 1 diabetes

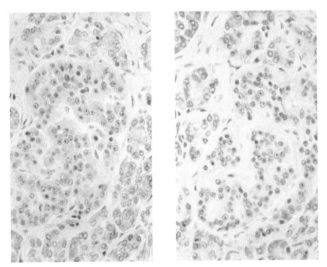

Figure 32 Autopsy section of an islet from a patient who had diabetes for 16 years. Although the islet looks fairly normal on H & E stain (left), insulin staining (right) shows it is devoid of β-cells

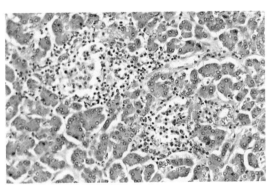

Figure 33 This is a section of pancreas from a 12-year-old boy who died of a cardiomyopathy. He had a family history of type 1 diabetes and was considered to be pre-diabetic because he had high titers of both insulin and islet cell autoantibodies in autopsy blood, but he did not have glycosuria in life. The photograph shows two islets affected by insulitis in his pancreas, confirming that immunologically mediated β-cell destruction takes place in the preclinical period of type 1 diabetes

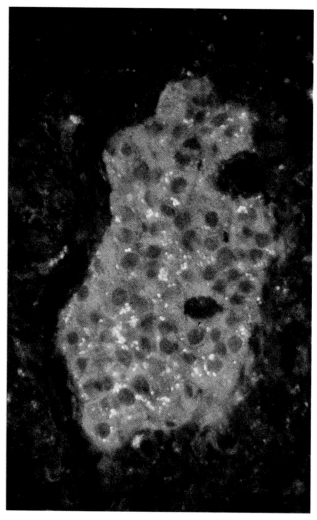

Figure 34 Circulating cytoplasmic islet-cell antibodies (ICA) can be found in most newly diagnosed type 1 diabetes mellitus (DM) patients, thereby providing evidence of an autoimmune pathogenesis of this disorder. ICA are also seen in the 'prediabetic' period and in siblings of type 1 DM patients, and are a marker of susceptibility to type 1 DM. This high-power view of a cryostat section of human pancreas was incubated with serum from a type 1 DM patient and stained by an indirect immunofluorescence technique using anti-human IgG fluorescinated antiserum. Although ICA are serologic markers of β-cell destruction, the antibodies also stain the entire islet, including glucagon and somatostatin cells (which, unlike the β-cells, are not destroyed). The positive reaction is confined to cell cytoplasm and the nuclei are unstained (seen as black dots)

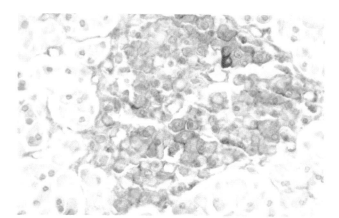

Figure 35 This section shows that all the endocrine cells (A, B, D, etc.) in this insulin-containing islet hyperexpress class 1 major histocompatibility complex (MHC). Note also that the islet is not inflamed (no lymphocytes). This suggests that hyperexpression of class 1 MHC precedes insulitis within any given islet and is not simply the result of secretion of cytokines by inflammatory cells in the insulitis infiltrate

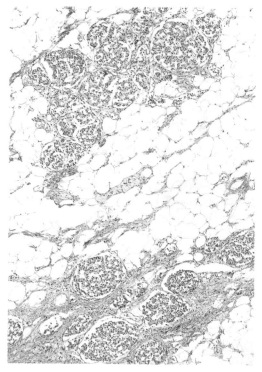

Figure 36 Glucose intolerance occurs in about 30% of cases of cystic fibrosis, although only 1–2% of patients have frank diabetes. This low-power view of the pancreas of a 14-year-old child with cystic fibrosis complicated by diabetes shows complete atrophy of the exocrine pancreas, but with survival of the islets. Some of the islets (lower part of field) are embedded in fibrous tissue. H & E

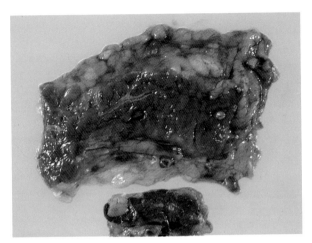

Figure 37 This is a coronal section of the tail of the pancreas from a patient with hemochromatosis. Note the brown color of the pancreas compared with the surrounding fat. Normal pancreas tissue appears pale. The smaller piece of pancreas has been stained with Prussian blue to show the presence of iron deposits

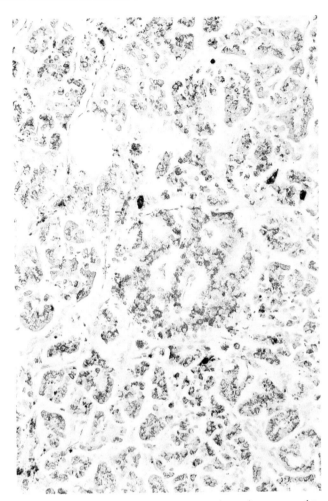

Figure 38 Hemochromatosis. Hemosiderin deposits in this low-power view of pancreas are stained blue. Note the accumulation of iron in the endocrine cells of the islet (center) as well as in the acinar cells of the exocrine pancreas. Prussian blue staining

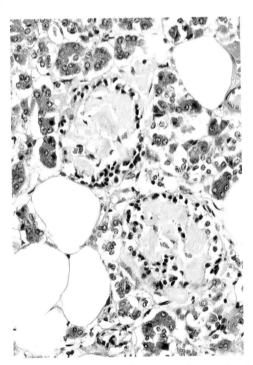

Figure 39 The characteristic histologic abnormality in type 2 diabetes mellitus (DM) is amyloid deposition in the islets, which is significant in around two-thirds of cases. Increasing amounts of amyloid deposition are associated with progressive islet cell damage, which probably contributes to the insulin deficiency of type 2 DM. In this pancreas from a patient who had type 2 DM of long standing, two islets containing large deposits of amorphous pink-staining amyloid can be seen

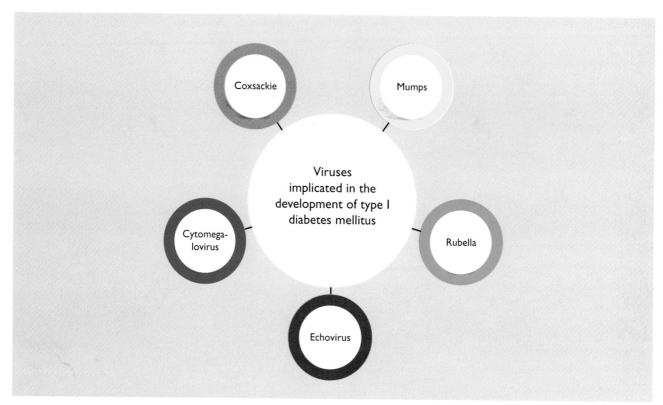

Figure 40 Viruses have been suggested to be a cause or factor in the development of type 1 diabetes mellitus (DM), and are thought to be the most likely agents to trigger the disease, probably on the basis of genetic predisposition, in some cases. Evidence comes from epidemiologic studies and the isolation of viruses from the pancreas of a few recently diagnosed type 1 DM patients. Mumps and Coxsackie viruses can cause acute pancreatitis, and Coxsackie virus can cause β-cell destruction

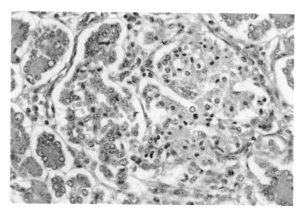

Figure 41 Autopsy sample of histology of Coxsackie B viral pancreatitis in a neonate. Coxsackie B viral infection may cause inflammatory destruction of the β-cells and Coxsackie B viruses have been isolated from the pancreas of patients with new-onset type 1 diabetes. Injection of such isolates into mice causes insulitis and β-cell damage. The similarity between this picture and the previous one of insulitis is obvious. Nevertheless, although Coxsackie B virus may be diabetogenic in men, its precise etiologic importance in the development of type 1 diabetes remains unclear

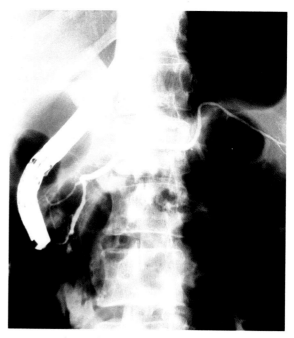

Figure 42 This endoscopic retrograde cholangiopancreatogram shows a normal pancreatic duct

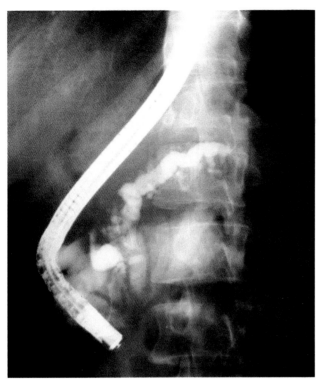

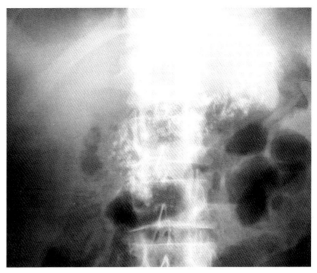

Figure 44 Plain abdominal radiograph showing pancreatic calcification due to chronic pancreatitis. Diabetes occurs in around 45% of cases of chronic pancreatitis and is usually mild. Approximately one-third of patients will ultimately require insulin treatment to maintain adequate glycemic control

Figure 43 This endoscopic retrograde cholangiopancreatogram shows the typical appearances of chronic pancreatitis. There is a dilated pancreatic duct with amputation and beading of the side branches

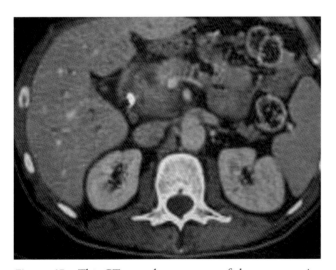

Figure 45 This CT scan shows cancer of the pancreas. An association between adenocarcinoma of the pancreas and diabetes has long been recognized. Pancreatic cancer may precede the diagnosis of diabetes, but some epidemiologic studies suggest that there is an increased risk of pancreatic cancer in diabetic patients. Unexplained weight loss or back pain in a patient with type 2 diabetes must always raise the suspicion of underlying pancreatic cancer

3   Treatment

DIETARY TREATMENT FOR TYPE I DIABETES MELLITUS

An integral component of diabetes management by both the health-care professional and the patient with diabetes is the need to know the principles of dietary management of the condition. Nutrition is complex and a registered dietician is best placed to offer advice on recommended diets, although all team members need to be knowledgeable about nutrition therapy. The dietary recommendations for patients with type 1 diabetes mellitus (DM) do not differ greatly from those recommended for the general population. Dietary advice must be tailored to the given patient and certain population groups require special consideration, for example, particular ethnic minorities or children.

The total fat intake should not exceed 30% of total energy intake, and < 10% should come from saturated fats. Dietary cholesterol intake should be less than 300 mg/day. Intake of trans unsaturated fatty acids should be kept to a minimum. Carbohydrates, predominantly complex carbohydrates, should comprise > 50% of the total energy intake. Foods containing carbohydrate from whole grains, fruits and vegetables should be included in the diet. The total amount of carbohydrate in meals or snacks is more important than the source, type or glycemic index of the carbohydrate. Non-nutritive sweeteners are safe when consumed within acceptable daily limits. Consumption of simple sugars, e.g. sucrose, is acceptable in moderate amounts, as they do not cause acute hyperglycemia (unlike glucose which does) as long as they are consumed within a healthy diet. Dietary fiber should be increased, ideally to > 30 g/day, and it is preferable that this be taken in the form of natural soluble fiber as found in legumes, grain cereals or fruit. Protein should comprise approximately 10–15% of total energy intake.

Moderate sodium restriction and the national general recommendations for alcohol ingestion should be followed, and 'diabetic foods' and 'diabetic beers' are best avoided. Regular main meals with between-meal and bedtime snacks remain the usual basis of dietary treatment for type 1 DM patients. The size and distribution of the meals should be dictated by the individual patient's preferences and habits, unless these give rise to major problems with glycemic control or weight gain.

An understanding of the carbohydrate content of foods remains necessary, but detailed and over-precise 'carbohydrate exchange lists' can be misleading. Although some centers have abandoned the use of formal carbohydrate exchange lists, others remain enthusiastic about their use to match insulin dose with quantity of carbohydrate ingested in an attempt to improve smooth blood glucose control and allow patients greater choice of food intake (see Dose Adjustment for Normal Eating program below).

One advantage to patients of the widely used basal-bolus insulin regimens is that meals no longer need to be taken at a fixed time to avoid hypoglycemia – a degree of flexibility is allowed by matching the bolus ingestion of rapidly acting insulin to the meal time.

DIETARY TREATMENT FOR TYPE 2 DIABETES MELLITUS

Diet is the cornerstone of treatment of type 2 DM. Simple initial advice for calorie restriction and avoidance of sweet foods and drinks can lead to symptomatic improvement and a fall in blood glucose levels before any reductions in body weight are detectable. More detailed advice is then required to formulate a long-term strategy. The main goal is to correct obesity as weight loss will improve blood glucose control, lower blood pressure and lower blood lipid concentrations, all of which may be expected to improve the prognosis for patients with type 2 DM. A diet similar to that advised for patients with type 1 DM is recommended with special emphasis on lowered fat intake and reduced energy intake.

Dietary failure is common in the treatment of overweight associated with type 2 DM. At the outset, avoidance of fat in the diet must be stressed and it is important to define realistic body-weight targets and rates of weight loss. Discussion of ideal body weight from actuarial tables is usually met with dismay and discourages patients. A rate of weight loss of about 0.5 kg/week is realistic. Progressive long-term weight loss is rarely achieved. Positive discussion and encouragement are to be recommended as outright censure and accusations of 'cheating' are unhelpful. The use of orlistat (Xenical®, Roche) which reduces intestinal fat absorption may help some patients with their weight loss program. An increase in regular exercise and avoidance of smoking are also advisable.

Exercise and diabetes

Taking exercise has been a recommendation in patients with type 2 DM for a very long time. The corollary is that type 2 DM is more likely to occur in populations that are physically sedentary. Thus, patients with type 2 DM may be innately resistant to the suggestion that they take physical exercise and this frequently presents a challenge to diabetes educators and physicians. From a meta-analysis of clinical trials examining the effect of exercise interventions on glycemic control and BMI in type 2 DM, subjects in the intervention group achieved a glycosylated hemoglobin (HbA_{1c}) value that was 0.66% lower than that of the control group. Interestingly, there was no difference in body weight between the exercise and the control group suggesting that exercise has a beneficial effect independent of a reduction in body weight.

An inverse association between mortality and physical activity has been demonstrated in men with type 1 DM. Regular exercise has also been shown to lead to reduced morbidity and mortality in type 2 DM. Furthermore, as discussed at more length elsewhere (*vida supra*), exercise has been shown to reduce the risk of developing type 2 diabetes in people with impaired glucose tolerance. Exercise improves insulin sensitivity in both those with impaired glucose tolerance and diabetes – both type 1 and type 2.

Specific recommendations and guidelines for exercise by diabetic patients have been published by the American Diabetes Association and it is important to stress that even non-strenuous exercise such as regular walking ('walking the malls') is beneficial. Prescriptions for exercise should be tailored to the individual patient taking into account comorbidity and patient choice. Patients are not likely to continue with sports or exercises that they do not enjoy – in practical terms this may create real problems for many patients and their advisors.

For patients with type 1 DM, a reduction in insulin dosage is often required before exercise with dose reductions of 30–50% being common, although individuals' response to exercise may differ and the necessary dose reduction has to be determined by trial and error using blood glucose measurements before, during and after exercise. It will also be affected by the type, duration and intensity of the physical activity. In type 2 DM, exercise does not usually cause hypoglycemia but may do so in those patients taking oral sulfonylureas or, of course, being treated with insulin. In normal subjects, insulin secretion declines during moderately intense aerobic exercise to compensate for increased muscle insulin sensitivity. In type 1 DM, as all insulin is exogenous, this cannot occur and this, in combination with increased insulin absorption if the insulin is injected into a limb which is subsequently exercised and the use of intermediate or long-acting insulin, often leads to hyperinsulinemia and hypoglycemia if corrective actions are not taken as indicated above. Paradoxically, if hypoinsulinemia occurs, especially during intensive exercise, increased glucose production, decreased peripheral glucose uptake and increased levels of counter-regulatory hormones leading to lipid breakdown and ketogenesis can cause the development of both hyperglycemia and ketosis.

INSULIN TREATMENT OF TYPE I DIABETES MELLITUS

The Diabetes Control and Complications Trial (DCCT) published in the USA in 1993 established beyond all reasonable doubt that intensive insulin therapy delays the onset and slows the progression of diabetic microvascular complications. The achievement of good blood glucose control while avoiding hypoglycemia is therefore the therapeutic goal for most patients with type 1 DM. For the majority of patients this proves to be a major challenge despite considerable input from the diabetic team. Diabetic specialist nurses have assumed a major role in helping patients reach appropriate targets.

A large number of insulins are available to treat patients with type 1 DM and many new formulations have appeared in recent years and continue to appear. Insulin analogs have rightly secured a firm place in the insulin market. For the non-specialist clinician it is advisable to become familiar with commonly prescribed insulins and the regimens that are applied in their use. In clinical practice, only two classes of insulin are needed in the attempt to mimic physiologic insulin secretion: a rapid-acting formulation to cover meals and a longer-acting preparation to provide steady state basal levels between meals and overnight. Rapid and longer-acting insulins can be combined in the same cartridge as a fixed mixture (or premixed insulins). Rapid-acting insulins include soluble (regular) insulin that should be injected around 30 min before a meal or rapid-acting insulin analogs (insulin lispro (Humalog®, Eli Lilly), insulin aspart (NovoRapid®, NovoNordisk) and insulin glulisine (Apidra®, Sanofi Aventis)) that can be injected at the time of the meal. Longer-acting insulin preparations include conventional NPH (isophane) insulin and the insulin analogs insulin glargine (Lantus®, Sanofi Aventis) and insulin detemir (Levemir®, NovoNordisk). In many countries, such as the UK, and more recently the USA, insulin delivery via a pen device, so called insulin pens, has become by far the most popular method of subcutaneous insulin administration. A list of commonly used insulin preparations is illustrated in Figure 50. Currently recommended insulin regimens are many and varied and include twice-daily insulins, basal-bolus regimens and continuous subcutaneous insulin infusion.

Twice-daily insulins – free or mixed

The simplest regimen is to inject insulin subcutaneously twice a day, before breakfast and before the evening meal. Although patients' needs differ, in general two-thirds of the total daily insulin dose is given in the morning with one-third in the evening. Using conventional insulin preparations, the ability of injections performed 30–40 min before meals to match postprandial glucose excursions, although crude, is illustrated in Figure 60. The ratio of soluble to isophane insulin can be determined by the patient's subsequent blood glucose measurements (with a starting ratio of one-third soluble to two-thirds isophane). Fine-tuning of the insulin doses is possible, however, many patients find this difficult and there is a place for the use of fixed mixtures that are available in many ratios of soluble to isophane (10/90, 20/80, 30/70, 40/60, 50/50). Pre-mixed insulins are widely used in analog form (Humalog Mix 25®, NovoMix 30®).

It is widely recognized that such regimens have their drawbacks. Inflexibility is one as is the need to eat three meals a day with mid-meal snacks to avoid hypoglycemia owing to the persistence of the effect of the short-acting insulin. In addition, the peak effect of the evening intermediate insulin occurs between midnight and 03.00 when the need is least and then diminishes towards morning when insulin requirements are rising again. Increasing the before-dinner isophane to cope with pre-breakfast hyperglycemia leads to nocturnal hypoglycemia which may go unrecognized and is one of the biggest problems in the treatment of type 1 DM. To some extent, this can be counteracted by delaying the evening injection of isophane insulin to before bed.

Basal-bolus regimens

This regimen has become perhaps the most widely used in recent years. The rationale is that a long-acting insulin administered at bedtime provides a 'basal' insulin level that is supplemented before meals by short-acting insulin to cope with the rise in postprandial blood glucose.

Earlier regimens most commonly used NPH (isophane) as the basal insulin but, more recently, NPH has been increasingly replaced by insulin glargine

(Lantus®) and insulin detemir (Levemir®). Glargine can be given at any fixed time of day most commonly before bed or at breakfast. These later insulins exhibit more reproducibility in terms of their biological action compared to NPH. Some regimens incorporate the use of twice-daily injections of glargine or detemir. A major advantage of such regimens is that they allow the patient more flexibility with the timing of meals; if lunch is delayed, for instance, the injection of short-acting insulin can simply be given later. Patients should not, however, be tempted to miss either meals or the preceding insulin.

Although allowing greater flexibility, there is no overwhelming evidence that the multiple-injection regimen produces better glycemic control than twice-daily injections of short-acting insulin with isophane.

The short-acting insulin analogs have much shorter onsets of action than soluble insulin and shorter durations of action. One major advantage to patients is that they may be injected at the time of eating rather than 30–40 min beforehand. Furthermore, evidence suggests that their usage may be associated with less hypoglycemia occurring mid-morning, mid-afternoon and during the night. These insulins have rapidly become immensely popular with diabetic patients, especially the young. Humalog has usefully been formulated into a fixed mixture preparation (Humalog Mix 25) with a short to intermediate ratio of 25/75 and NovoRapid into a fixed mixture (NovoMix 30) with a short to intermediate ratio of 30/70.

There has been much debate regarding the importance of insulin species, centered on the hypothesis that the use of human insulin (produced by either enzymatic modification or recombinant-DNA technology) is associated with lack of hypoglycemia awareness. The hypothesis has tended to be patient-driven and the current consensus, based on a wealth of clinical studies, is that there is no scientific evidence to support such a contention. However, if patients express a wish to resume porcine insulin, they should be allowed to do so as no harm will result from such a switch.

Continuous subcutaneous insulin infusion

Continuous subcutaneous insulin infusion (CSII) attempts to emulate physiologic insulin secretion with low basal insulin delivery using a small portable battery-driven pump and a reservoir of short-acting soluble insulin. From the pump, a plastic delivery cannula that ends in a fine-gauge 'butterfly' needle is usually inserted subcutaneously into the anterior abdominal wall. The site of implantation must be changed every 1–2 days to avoid local inflammation. The basal infusion is supplemented at mealtimes by a prandial boost activated by the patient. The basal rate and prandial boosts are determined according to each individual patient after a brief admission to hospital or by intensive outpatient education.

Continuous subcutaneous insulin requires a comprehensive education program prior to its use. The hospitals participating in the use of this technique are required to provide a 24-h telephone service so that pump patients can receive immediate advice.

Most patients using this method of treatment achieve excellent control of blood glucose levels. However, disadvantages include the logistic problems in setting up such a service, the problem of funding the pumps which are expensive and the possibility of system malfunction, usually related to the insulin syringe in the pump, cannula, needle or infusion site. Such problems may partly explain the incidence of ketoacidosis in patients treated by continuous subcutaneous insulin, although many experienced centers throughout the world are now reporting a significant decrease in ketoacidosis rates. Skin complications are also seen, but hypoglycemia is no more common than with conventional treatments despite the ability of CSII to produce a significant improvement in blood glucose control. At present, the use of insulin pumps should be considered for selected patients (such as, when conventional insulin injection treatment has failed with poor glycemic control, unstable blood glucose levels and significant recurrent hypoglycemia) and requires referral to centers specializing in this treatment modality. Increasing numbers of patients without any of the specific problems outlined above may opt for this form of treatment if appropriate funding is available and CSII usage is particularly high in the USA and certain countries of the European Union where such funding is available.

BLOOD GLUCOSE MONITORING

The ability of the diabetic patient to monitor the effect of their treatment on their blood glucose levels remains one of the major challenges of diabetes care.

At long last exciting new methodology appears to be on the horizon. At present, however, most patients self-monitor their blood glucose using a wide array of commercially available blood glucose meters which all achieve clinically acceptable standards of accuracy and precision at least in laboratory assessment. Not all patients (nor indeed nurses and doctors in hospital wards) are able to achieve such standards. This emphasizes the need for adequate instruction in the technique and regular quality-control assessment. Unfortunately, finger pricking to produce an aliquot of blood for self-monitoring is an unpleasant procedure, certainly associated with more discomfort than insulin injections. This may inhibit the performance of testing using current technology.

Blood glucose measurements are taken before and after meals and, on the basis of a profile of several days' readings, a decision is made regarding the need to alter the insulin dosages. In practice, however, although most patients become reasonably adept at blood glucose measurement, only a minority of patients acquire the skill of appropriate adjustment of insulin dosages. The exception to this seems to be most patients who have been on a DAFNE course as alluded to below.

Furthermore, there is controversy as to the minimum number of readings required each day. A compromise would be two readings per day with variations in the timing of the readings on alternate days. Alternatively profiles of four or more readings may be done on selected days during the week. More intensive monitoring is recommended during intercurrent illness and when insulin treatment is being changed or adjusted.

Among the more tangible benefits of self-monitoring are that the technique allows patients to recognize that certain symptoms represent hypoglycemia and that the ingestion of certain foods leads to an unacceptable increase in blood glucose concentration. It also allows the assessment of the individual's glucose response to various types of exercise. There is no conclusive evidence of benefit of self-monitoring of blood glucose in patients with type 2 diabetes except for those on insulin therapy, although, it may be helpful during concurrent illness.

Clearly recognized disadvantages of current blood glucose sampling systems are the need for skin lancing and the practical limitations of obtaining samples frequently enough to allow meaningful manipulation of insulin dosage with either subcutaneous injections or continuous pump methods. Technological progress has been made here in the development and availability of continuous glucose monitoring using a subcutaneously implanted continuous monitoring system (MiniMed Inc., Sylmar, CA, USA). The subcutaneous sensor is connected by a cable to a monitor/microprocessor device that is worn externally (Figure 69). Interstitial fluid glucose is measured frequently and the data are downloaded at a later time. This information can then be used to refine and adjust patients' diabetes management resulting in improved glycemic control and avoidance of hypoglycemia. Studies to date have demonstrated disturbing changes in blood glucose values that could not have been anticipated using conventional self-monitoring techniques. A wristwatch-like device that uses a process known as reverse iontophoresis and is able to produce similar results on a real-time basis with warning of hypoglycemia has been marketed, but has not proved to be as useful and as acceptable in practice as had been thought at product launch.

ROLE OF EDUCATION

Most type 1 DM patients achieve, at best, only suboptimal control of blood glucose levels. Around 25% of adult type 1 diabetic patients exhibit persistent poor glycemic control. Lower socioeconomic status and psychologic factors including lack of motivation, emotional distress, depression and eating disorders have been associated with poor control. Clinical experience over decades and data from the Diabetes Control and Complications Trial (DCCT) emphasize the role of diabetic education in the attainment of good glycemic control. Constant teaching, encouragement and support of these patients combined with open access to diabetes specialist nurses (DSNs) are fundamental to this goal. Methods of improving glycemic control include strategies that facilitate self-management, such as motivational strategies, coping-orientated education and psychosocial therapies, and intensification of insulin injection therapy or CSII. One self-empowering intensive educational program called DAFNE (Dose Adjustment for Normal Eating) originally developed in Germany has consistently been shown to lead to an improved quality of life, greater freedom of choice of food and a fall in HbA$_{1c}$ levels.

This program has been taken up enthusiastically in many centers.

However, there are patients who remain supremely resistant to such measures. Patients with major metabolic instability, referred to as 'brittle' diabetics, are usually young women who are mildly overweight and who tend to spend several weeks each year in hospital. Although there are many theories as to the cause of such brittleness, for example, defective insulin absorption or inappropriate insulin regimens, there is a growing conviction that psychologic disturbance is the root cause. Not unexpectedly, motivation appears to be a key factor in achieving good blood glucose control. This is best exemplified in cases of diabetic pregnancy where virtually all mothers-to-be manage to achieve near normoglycemia.

ASSESSMENT OF GLYCEMIC CONTROL

The concept of diabetic control includes a feeling of well-being, avoidance of hypoglycemia and absence of ketoacidosis. It must also include an assessment of blood glucose levels. As mentioned above, a false assessment of the degree of control established can be made if this only includes the patient's own blood results. Measurement of HbA_{1c} or total HbA_1 must also be included when assessing control and is complementary to the patient's results. Normal self-monitored blood glucose results in the presence of elevated HbA_{1c} usually imply either falsification of results, an inability to perform the test properly or a fault in the blood glucose meter, if one is being used.

Glycosylated (glycated) hemoglobin refers to a series of minor hemoglobin components formed by the adduction of glucose to normal adult hemoglobin. The usefulness of this measurement is that it reflects the integrated blood glucose concentration over a period that approximates the half-life of the red cell, 6–8 weeks. Although factors which affect red cell survival may invalidate this test, they are uncommon in clinical practice (except perhaps in patients of African-Caribbean origin).

Although measurement of HbA_{1c} has become the gold standard in the assessment of diabetic control it may not accurately reflect the true level of excursions of glucose in the period studied. What HbA_{1c} level should patients try to attain? Ideally, the answer is normality, but this is a counsel of perfection that may be associated with an unacceptably high risk of hypoglycemia. Levels of around 6% are certainly acceptable and patients should probably strive to maintain levels of $\leq 7\%$. It is important to know the normal ranges for different laboratories (depending on the methodology used for measurement) before making comparisons between clinical centers. Ideally the normal range for HbA_{1c} should be DCCT aligned.

Integrated glycemia over a much shorter period of time may be assessed by measurement of glycated proteins (fructosamine), although, because of uncertainty pertaining to its use, this assay has not become widely adopted.

DRUG AND INSULIN TREATMENT FOR TYPE 2 DIABETES MELLITUS

The treatment of type 2 DM continues to be a major therapeutic challenge. Our knowledge of the efficacy of treatment strategies was informed by the landmark intervention study, the United Kingdom Prospective Diabetes Study (UKPDS). In this study, an intensive glucose control policy, which was able to maintain a HbA_{1c} value 0.9% lower than conventional treatment, was associated with significant reductions in the risk of microvascular endpoints. The UKPDS has demonstrated the progressive nature of type 2 diabetes and the need to employ combination treatments and insulin to achieve target goals. Redefining of such goals has also occurred, and the American Diabetes Association has proposed a target value for HbA_{1c} of 7.0%, while the European Diabetes Project Group has proposed a HbA_{1c} value of $\leq 6.5\%$.

Dietary modification and physical activity are the mainstay of treatment of type 2 diabetes. However, it is well recognized that only a minority of type 2 diabetes patients are able to achieve long-term glycemic control by such measures alone. Failure of dietary treatment is due to either (or both) an inability to sustain the necessary diet modifications or worsening of the diabetic state. Drug treatment should not be instituted until an adequate trial of diet has been shown to have failed. However, there is now an increasing tendency to advocate an intensive aggressive therapeutic strategy from the outset to reduce fasting blood glucose and HbA_{1c} levels to those defined above in an effort to minimize the risk of future complications. When diet fails, treatment with oral hypoglycemic agents is indicated, initially as monotherapy, and if and when that fails as combination therapy. Five classes of oral antidiabetic agents are currently available. In the past sulfonylureas have been widely prescribed as first-line agents after dietary failure (in some countries α-glucosidase inhibitors have had this role). However, the UKPDS has shown significant benefits for metformin as a first-line agent especially in obese patients. The place of agents such as meglitinides and thiazolidinediones (glitazones) as initial monotherapy is still subject to assessment and review.

Sulfonylureas

Sulfonylureas stimulate insulin secretion from the β-cell. They also appear to sensitize the β-cell to various other insulin secretagogs, such as glucose. An improvement in insulin resistance may also be observed with the sulfonylureas, but this is thought to be secondary to their primary mode of action and not a direct effect of the drug.

Among sulfonylureas, there is a wide variation in half-life, ranging from 3–8 h (tolbutamide) to 35 h (chlorpropamide). Side-effects, such as skin rashes, are relatively uncommon with the exception of hypoglycemia. Particular caution should be taken in type 2 diabetic patients with renal failure. Sulfonylureas have a tendency to produce weight gain, although any intervention that improves diabetic control in a patient following an isocaloric diet would be expected to result in such an effect.

Metformin

Metformin lowers plasma glucose by inhibiting hepatic glucose production and increasing the sensitivity of peripheral tissue to insulin. It does not usually cause hypoglycemia but, as it is renally excreted, it should not be used in patients with renal impairment.

Gastrointestinal side-effects are common and include diarrhea, anorexia, dyspepsia and a metallic taste in the mouth. To minimize the occurrence of side-effects, patients should be started on a low dose. Weight gain is usually not a problem with metformin, possibly because it has a slight anorectic effect. Lactic acidosis (which led to the withdrawal of phenformin) is a potentially serious side-effect of metformin therapy, but is rare and unlikely to occur if the drug is not used in patients with hepatic disease, renal impairment or severe cardiac problems.

α-Glucosidase inhibitors

These drugs, which include acarbose (Glucobay®, Bayer) and miglitol (Glyset®, Bayer), are widely used first-line agents in Japan. They delay the absorption of complex carbohydrates from the gastrointestinal tract and are of value in controlling postprandial hyperglycemia; however, their blood glucose lowering effect is lower than those of metformin or the sulfonylureas, and the side-effects of flatulence and diarrhea often limit their tolerability.

Meglitinides (or prandial glucose regulators)

These newer agents, like the sulfonylureas, act via closure of K-ATP channels in the β-cells, although their receptor binding characteristics are different. They include repaglinide (NovoNorm®, Novo Nordisk) and nateglinide (Starlix®, Novartis) and they rapidly produce a short-lived insulin release that is dependent on the concentration of glucose. Thus, taken before meals they restore towards normal the delayed and impaired insulin response to meals seen in type 2 diabetes, without causing hypoglycemia. Evidence suggests that prandial glucose spikes may have a role in the development of diabetic macrovascular complications but, as yet, there is no consensus as to the place of prandial glucose regulation in the management of type 2 diabetes. Meglitinides may safely be used in combination with metformin. In some countries, the enthusiasm for use of these drugs appears to be declining and they have not established themselves as first-line agents. The cost of meglitinides is high compared with that of generic sulfonylureas.

Thiazolidinediones (glitazones)

The initial enthusiasm for the thiazolidinediones (or glitazones) was tempered by the severe hepatotoxicity associated with troglitazone, which has now been withdrawn. The newer glitazones, rosiglitazone (Avandia®, GlaxoSmithKline) and pioglitazone (Actos®, Takeda) show no significant association with hepatotoxicity. Their mode of action is mediated by activation of the nuclear receptor peroxisome proliferator-activated receptor-gamma (PPARγ), which is found predominantly in adipose tissue but also in skeletal muscle and liver. This leads to stimulation of insulin-sensitive proteins with a reduction of hepatic glucose production and an increase in peripheral glucose uptake. Thiazolidinediones act to increase fatty acid uptake into adipocytes thus lowering triglyceride and non-esterified fatty acid levels which contribute to the favorable effect on glucose metabolism outlined above. They also induce adipocyte differentiation. As monotherapy these agents are comparable with sulfonylureas and metformin but, because of the effects outlined above, they may prove to have a particularly beneficial role in ameliorating insulin resistance. They reduce intra-abdominal fat deposition but also promote peripheral fat deposition. This latter effect and their tendency to produce edema is associated with weight gain. They should not be used in patients with cardiac failure or who are at risk of developing heart failure.

In a prospective randomized controlled trial (the PROACTIVE study), 5238 patients with type 2 DM who had evidence of macrovascular disease were assigned to pioglitazone or placebo and studied for nearly 36 months. Although there was no statistically significant reduction in the study composite primary endpoint, the use of pioglitazone was associated with a significant reduction in the secondary composite endpoint of all-cause mortality, non-fatal myocardial infarction and stroke, suggesting that glitazones may have a role in secondary prevention of macrovascular events in patients with type 2 diabetes.

Insulin

If diabetic control remains unacceptable despite dietary improvements with oral drug treatment, insulin therapy may be indicated. Insulin is the only efficacious therapy in type 2 DM once significant β-cell failure has supervened. Oral agents fail to lower blood glucose levels adequately once β-cell reserve falls below about 15% of normal. Approximately half of all patients with type 2 DM will need insulin therapy within 6 years of diagnosis because of a progressive decline in β-cell function. It seems sensible to outline this potential future therapeutic direction to patients at the time of diagnosis. In patients with type 2 DM, insulin therapy may be associated with an increase in weight, especially in those who are over eating in the first place. This is unavoidable as the patients are unlikely, at this stage, to reduce their caloric intake. If substantially improved glycemic control is obtained, this will probably override the detrimental effects of any weight gained by the patient. However, the majority of normal-weight or moderately overweight type 2 DM patients transferring to insulin gain only a modest amount of weight (around 2–4 kg).

There are many ways of giving insulin to patients with type 2 DM and each regimen has its own advocates. No universal consensus exists, although studies examining this issue are in progress. One simple and popular approach is to give a subcutaneous injection of an intermediate or long-acting insulin (NPH, insulin glargine or insulin detemir) before bed with the object of normalizing the pre-breakfast blood glucose. Possible alternative regimens, or when the above approach fails to deliver adequate glycemic control, include twice-daily injections of fixed mixtures of soluble and intermediate-acting insulins (e.g. Human Mixtard 30, NovoMix 30 (Novo Nordisk) or Humalog Mix 25 (Eli Lilly)) given before or at breakfast and the evening meal according to insulin type. Finally, and especially in the context of severe insulin deficiency, insulin may be administered in a basal bolus regimen, as for type 1 DM patients, with short-acting insulin given with each meal accompanied by an injection of a longer-acting insulin before bed. Metformin treatment can be continued in those who are overweight to lower insulin resistance. In the USA, thiazolidinediones (glitazones) are licensed for use in combination with insulin except in those who show any evidence of heart failure. Such a combination is not yet licensed in Europe. Insulin therapy dictates the need to practice self blood glucose monitoring.

Other drugs

Logically, drugs used for the treatment of obesity might have a beneficial effect in type 2 DM by improving insulin sensitivity as a result of weight loss. Studies have demonstrated such benefit for the lipase inhibitor orlistat (Xenical) and for the serotonin–norepinephrine reuptake inhibitor sibutramine (Knoll Pharmaceuticals), but the exact role of these drugs in the management of type 2 DM is not clear.

Treatment strategy

Metformin is the drug of choice in overweight patients who are not intolerant of this agent. In those overweight patients who are intolerant of metformin, glitazone monotherapy is a possible alternative. In patients who are not overweight (BMI 19–25 or 19–23 in South Asian people), metformin or a sulfonylurea can be used. When monotherapy fails, a second drug is added, e.g. a sulfonylurea or glitazone for those on metformin alone or metformin or a glitazone for those on a sulfonylurea alone. When treatment with two oral hypoglycemic agents fails then consideration should be given to the addition of insulin or the use of 'triple therapy' (sulfonylurea, metformin and a glitazone). In the regimens described a prandial glucose regulator may be substituted for a sulfonylurea, although a generic sulfonylurea would be preferred. As mentioned previously, some specialists use a glitazone in combination with insulin in special circumstances. If patients have a BMI of less than 19 at presentation they should be treated with a sulfonylurea but very frequently monitored as they may need to proceed to insulin therapy on an early basis.

No treatment of type 2 DM should focus solely on glycemic control. As the cause of death in type 2 DM is major vascular disease, rigorous attention must be paid to the treatment of hypertension, lowering of blood lipids, the cessation of smoking and an active program of exercise.

ISLET CELL AND PANCREATIC TRANSPLANTATION

The dream of every patient with type 1 DM is to permanently rid themselves of the need to administer exogenous insulin on a daily basis. Islet cell and pancreatic transplantation has the potential to achieve this aim.

Islet cell transplantation

The concept of transplanting pieces or extracts of pancreas in patients with diabetes is over a century old. By the 1980s, reports of successful allogeneic islet transplantation with the use of conventional immunosuppression and purified human islets from cadaveric donors began to appear. However, the overall rates of success internationally were reported to be less than 10%. In 2000, Shapiro and co-workers in Edmonton reported a 100% success rate in seven patients. The Edmonton patients were highly selected and a novel steroid-free immunosuppression regimen was used consisting of pre- and post-transplant daclizumab (an anti-interleukin 2 receptor monoclonal antibody), maintenance sirolimus and low-dose tacrolimus. An adequate mass of freshly isolated islets usually from two sequential donors was freshly transplanted by embolization into the liver through a small catheter placed under fluoroscopic guidance into the main portal vein. In an extended series of 32 consecutive patients with type 1 DM treated in Edmonton, the 1-year rate of sustained insulin independence was 85%. At present, the Edmonton protocol, or variants thereof, is being subjected to trials at several other international centers, with some centers already reporting successful cases. Clearly, there are many hurdles to overcome before islet cell transplantation can be a more universal technique not least of which is the skill in preparing the islets and the availability of donor pancreases.

Whole-pancreas transplantation

Until the advent of successful islet cell transplantation, whole-pancreas transplantation was the only technique that could consistently restore endogenous secretion of insulin responsive to normal mechanisms of feedback control. Many thousand (over 15 000 up to 2001) pancreatic transplantations have been performed worldwide, the majority of which have been simultaneous pancreas-kidney transplants (SPKs). Some centers, for example the Minnesota group, have been enthusiastic advocates of pancreas transplants alone (PTA) for selected patients. Surgical techniques have improved greatly over the past few decades and have incorporated both enteric and bladder drainage of the exocrine pancreas. Significant advances in immunosuppressive regimens, particularly with the introduction of the use of tacrolimus as an immunosuppressant, have contributed to better outcomes for transplanted patients. For SPK recipients the actuarial survival of patients and of functional pancreas grafts with complete independence from insulin are 94% and 89% at 1 year and 81% and 67% at 5 years, respectively. The results for PTA grafts remain inferior to SPK grafts with pancreas graft survival being significantly lower.

SPK remains an excellent treatment option for diabetic patients in advanced renal failure, while PTA may transform the lives of those with rapidly advancing microvascular complications or serious hypoglycemic unawareness, although life-long immunosuppression will remain an issue. Undoubtedly, further progress will be made especially with regard to immunosuppressive regimens; however, the problem of a shortage of cadaver organs will always exist, although some centers have employed the use of living donor segmental pancreas transplants.

It is speculated that further success with islet cell transplantation may reduce the need for SPK or PTA transplantation and improved diabetes treatments may obviate the need for both.

BIBLIOGRAPHY

Alberti KGGM, Gries FA. Management of non-insulin dependent diabetes in Europe: a consensus view. Diabetic Med 1988; 5: 275–81

American Diabetes Association. Nutritional recommendations and principles for people with diabetes mellitus. Diabetes Care 2000; 23 (Suppl I): s43–6

American Diabetes Association. Nutritional principles and recommendations in diabetes. Diabetes Care 2004; 27 (Suppl 1): s36–s46

DeVries JH, Snoek FJ, Heine RJ. Persistent poor glycaemic control in adult type 1 diabetes. A closer look at the problem. Diabetic Med 2004; 21: 1263–8

Dormandy JA, Charbonnel B, Eckland DJA, et al. Secondary prevention of macrovascular events in patients with type 2 diabetes in the PROactive Study (PROspective pioglitAzone Clinical Trial in macroVascular Events): a randomized controlled trial. Lancet 2005; 366: 1279–89

European IDDM Policy Group. Consensus guidelines for the management of insulin-dependent (type I) diabetes. Bussum: Medicom Europen BV, 1993

Gale EA. New hypoglycemic therapies. J R Coll Physicians Lond 2000; 34: 250–3

Gerich JE. Oral hypoglycaemic agents. N Engl J Med 1989; 34: 1231–45

Lebovitz HE, Banerji MA. Insulin resistance and its treatment by thiazolidinediones. Recent Prog Horm Res 2001; 56: 265–94

Mudaliar S, Henry RR. New oral therapies for type 2 diabetes mellitus: the glitazones or insulin sensitizers. Annu Rev Med 2001; 52: 239–57

Nutrition Subcommittee of the British Diabetic Association's Professional Advisory Committee. Dietary recommendations for people with diabetes: an update for the 1990s. Diabet Med 1992; 9: 189–202

Robertson PR. Islet transplantation as a treatment for diabetes – a work in progress. N Engl J Med 2004; 350: 694–705

Robertson RP, Davis C, Larsen J, et al. Pancreas and islet transplantation for patients with diabetes. Diabetes Care 2000; 23: 112–16

Shapiro AM, Lakey JR, Ryan EA, et al. Islet transplantation in seven patients with type I diabetes mellitus using a glucocorticoid-free immunosuppressive regimen. N Engl J Med 2000; 343: 230–8

Shapiro JAM, Ryan EA, Paty BW, Lakey JRT. Pancreas and islet transplantation. In Pickup J, Williams G, eds. Textbook of Diabetes, 3rd edn, Oxford: Blackwell Scientific Publications, 2003: 72.1–72.18

Sutherland DER, Gruessner RWG, Dunn DL, et al. Lessons learned from more than 1000 pancreas transplants at a single institution. Ann Surg 2001; 233: 463–501

Sutherland DER, Gruessner RWG, Gruessner AC. Pancreas transplantation for treatment of diabetes mellitus. World J Surg 2001; 25: 487–96

Tattersall RB, Gale EAM, eds. Diabetes; Clinical Management. Edinburgh: Churchill Livingstone, 1990

UK Prospective Diabetes Study (UKPDS) Group. Intensive blood-glucose control with sulphonylureas or insulin compared with conventional treatment and risk of complications in patients with type 2 diabetes (UKPDS 33). Lancet 1998; 352: 837–53

UK Prospective Diabetes Study (UKPDS) Group. Effect of intensive blood-glucose control with metformin on complications in overweight patients with type 2 diabetes (UKPDS 34). Lancet 1998; 352: 854–65

Yki-Jarvinen H. Combination therapies with insulin in type 2 diabetes. Diabetes Care 2001; 24: 758–67

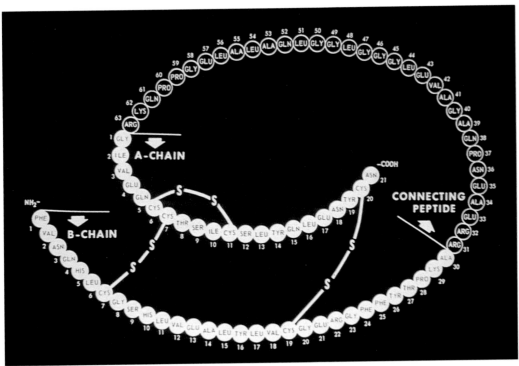

Figure 46 Proinsulin. Insulin is produced in the β-cells of the islets of Langerhans by cleavage of the precursor proinsulin into insulin and C-peptide. Measurement of C-peptide, especially following intravenous injection of 1 mg of glucagon, is a useful indicator of β-cell function as C-peptide and insulin are secreted in equimolar amounts and the former is minimally extracted by the liver. This test can be used to differentiate between types 1 and 2 diabetes mellitus in cases of diagnostic confusion

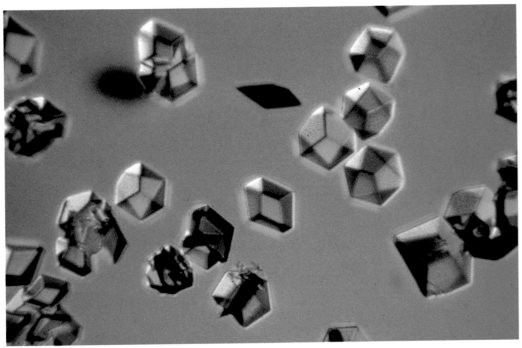

Figure 47 Insulin crystals. Insulin is stored in β-cells as hexamers complexed with zinc. Insulin–zinc hexamers readily form crystals which are stored in the pancreatic granules. In the blood, insulin is not seen in aggregated forms such as dimers or hexamers, but as monomers which are formed when insulin granules are liberated

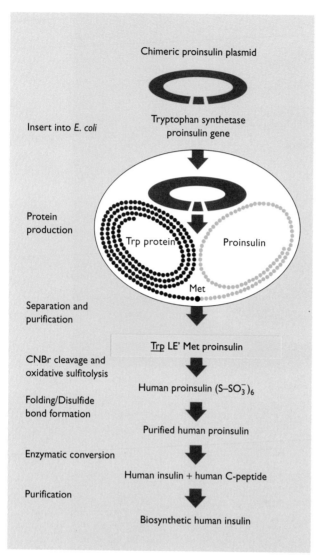

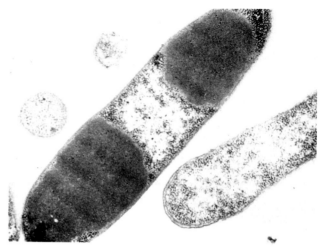

Figure 49 *Escherichia coli* distended by biosynthetic human proinsulin before lysis

Figure 48 Insulin for therapeutic use was previously produced solely from porcine or bovine sources. Human insulin is now manufactured by two different processes: enzymatic conversion of porcine to human insulin; and biosynthesis of human insulin. Porcine and human insulin differ only in a single residue at the C terminus of the β chain. Enzymatic conversion involves substitution of the porcine B30 alanine residue by threonine to produce the semisynthetic human insulin 'emp' (enzymatically modified porcine). The biosynthesis of human insulin using recombinant-DNA technology involves insertion of a synthetic gene coding for human proinsulin into a bacterial plasmid, which is then introduced into a bacterium such as *Escherichia coli*. Ultimately, the synthetic gene is transcribed in quantity and its messenger RNA translated into proinsulin

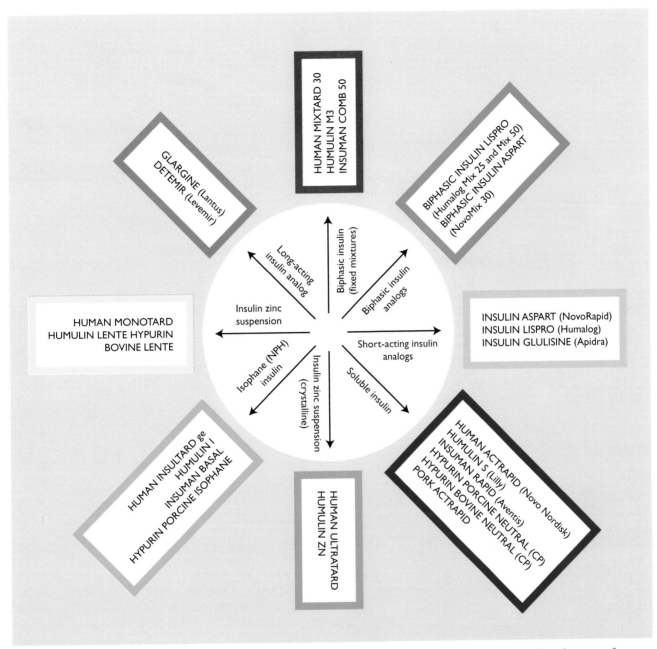

Figure 50 Over 300 insulin preparations are available worldwide. They may be classified according to their duration of action: short-acting (soluble, neutral or regular), intermediate-acting (isophane), long-acting (insulin–zinc suspensions), and fixed mixtures of short- and intermediate-acting (biphasic insulins). Some of the most commonly used insulins are summarized in this figure. It is preferable for the non-specialist to become familiar with a small number of appropriate insulins and insulin regimens rather than attempt to know them all

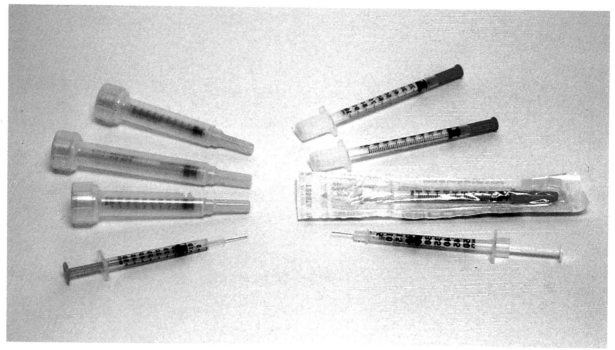

Figure 51 Modern plastic insulin syringes carry integral fixed needles and are designed to minimize dead space. Recent advances in needle manufacturing have resulted in very fine needles, which have greatly reduced the discomfort of insulin injection. Patients usually use the same syringe and needle for several injections

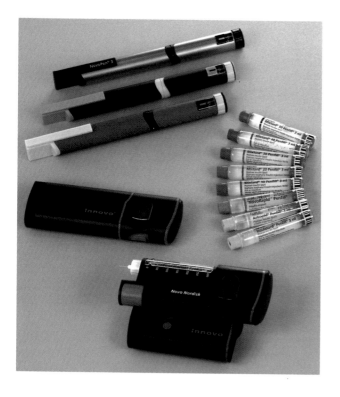

Figure 52 Illustrated here are the Novopen® 3 Classic and two Novopen Fun insulin pens with an assortment of 3 ml insulin cartridges, which are inserted into the pens. Such pens are now the most popular method of administering insulin. Originally developed for multiple-dose regimens using short-acting soluble insulin, they are now available with cartridges of intermediate-acting isophane or fixed mixtures of insulins for injection twice-daily. The particular advantages of these pens are convenience, speed and ease of injection as well as less pain owing to the development of very fine tipped needles. Disposable insulin pens are also available. Also shown is the Innovo® insulin doser device that allows the patient to dial-up the correct dose of insulin and displays the previous dose and the time passed since its delivery

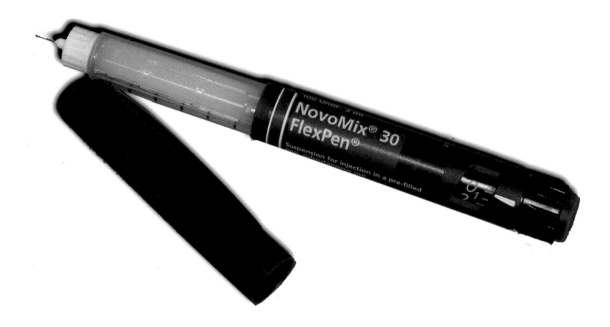

Figure 53 Insulin pens with preloaded cartridges are a popular method of insulin administration. The Flexpen® is one such pen and is a 3 ml preloaded delivery device for NovoMix® 30 and NovoRapid® insulins. It has tactile markings on the dose delivery button

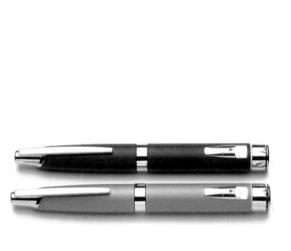

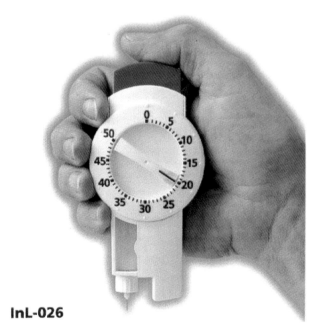

InL-026

Figure 54 The Humapen® Luxura insulin pen which has just been released exemplifies the user-friendly convenience of modern insulin pens which can be fitted into a jacket pocket or handbag

Figure 55 This novel pre-filled disposable device (Innolet®) has a plastic palm-held doser with a large 'egg-timer like' dial for dosing and is particularly useful for diabetic patients with hand problems or visual impairment

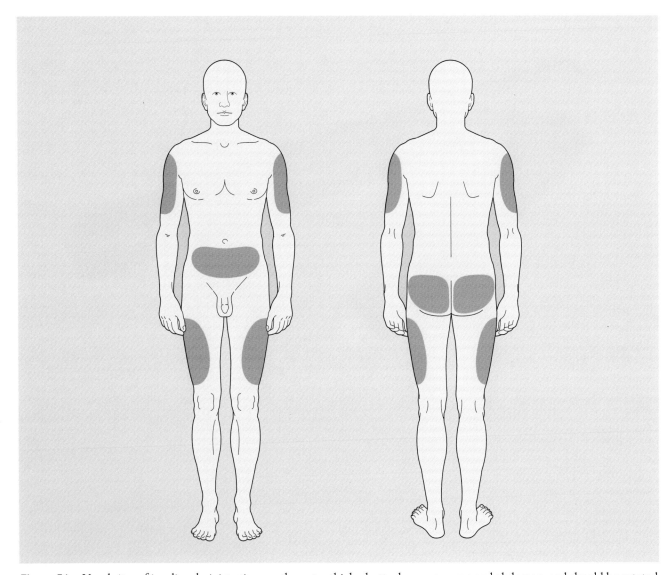

Figure 56   Usual sites of insulin administration are the outer thighs, buttocks, upper arms and abdomen, and should be rotated within each anatomic area as injection into exactly the same site may cause lipid hypertrophy (see Figure 64), which may hinder insulin absorption. Insulin absorption may vary from one site to another

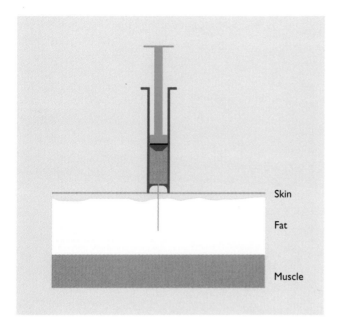

Figure 57 Insulin injection technique: the modern practice is to insert the needle vertically into the subcutaneous tissue. Needles of 8 mm in length are used with a pinch-up technique except in obese patients, in whom the standard 12-mm needle should be used. When insulin is being injected without pinch-up into the arms, 6-mm needles are recommended. It is no longer considered necessary to swab the skin with alcohol or to withdraw the skin plunger to check for blood. Care must be taken in thin patients to avoid intramuscular injection as this will result in more rapid absorption of insulin

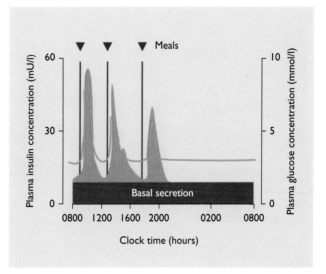

Figure 58 Physiologic plasma insulin and glucose profiles: in non-diabetic subjects, basal fasting insulin secretion is very low and suppresses hepatic glucose production, but meal ingestion results in a rapid increase in insulin secretion (shown here). This tight regulation keeps plasma glucose concentrations within a narrow range of about 3.5–7.5 mmol/l (63–135 mg/dl). It is this pattern which exogenous insulin therapy attempts to emulate

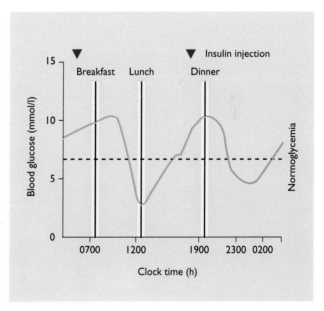

Figure 59 Effect of twice-daily subcutaneous injections of soluble insulin. Because soluble insulin has a peak effect 2–4 h after injection and a total duration of effect of 8–10 h, this regimen on its own cannot adequately control glucose; blood glucose concentrations will rise before the time of the next injection

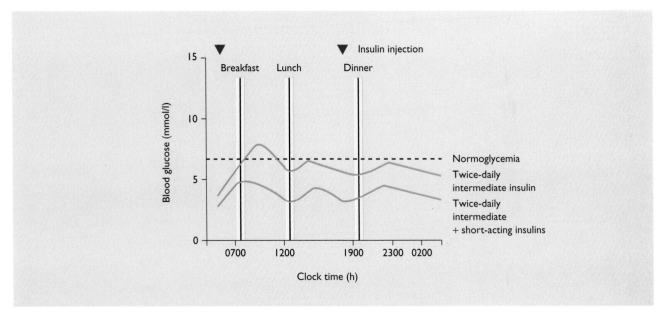

Figure 60 Effect of adding twice-daily soluble insulin injections to a regimen based on twice-daily intermediate-acting (isophane) insulin. Many newly presenting type 1 diabetes mellitus patients who have residual endogenous insulin secretion can be controlled with twice-daily isophane, two-thirds in the morning and one-third in the evening. However, if postprandial hyperglycemia is pronounced, soluble insulin can be added to one or both injections. Alternatively, fixed mixtures of soluble insulin and isophane can be tried

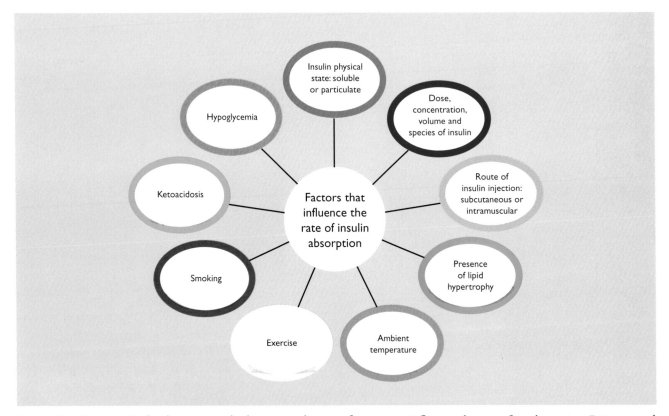

Figure 61 Once insulin has been injected subcutaneously, many factors may influence the rate of its absorption. Patients need to be made aware of this as such factors may occasionally explain erratic diabetic control

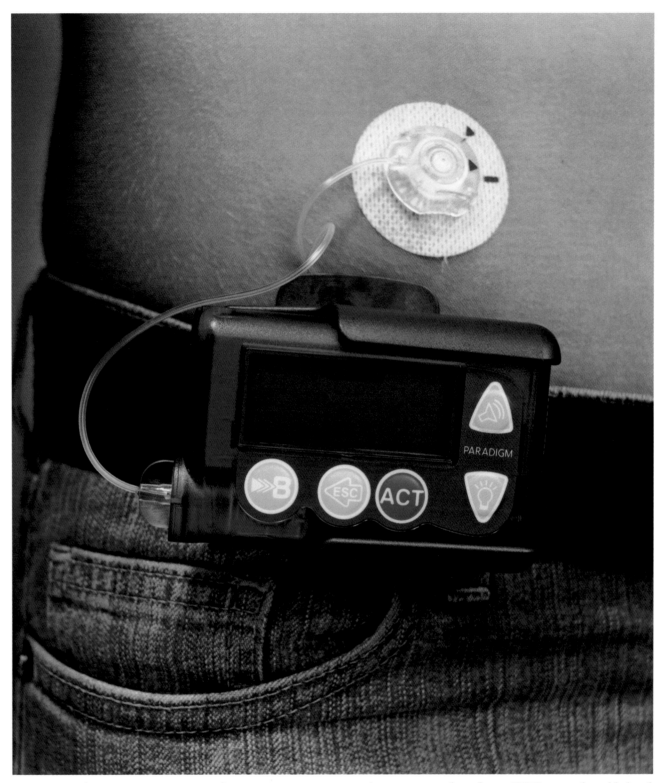

Figure 62   This patient is wearing an infuser to receive continuous subcutaneous insulin infusion (CSII) as an adjustable basal rate of insulin delivery augmented at mealtimes by patient-activated boosts. Patients employing CSII must have access to comprehensive education on its use, and to centers which can provide supervision by experienced staff and a 24-h telephone service for advice. Long-term strict control of blood glucose levels can be achieved, but this regimen is not without its problems; death may occur owing to sudden ketoacidosis if the insulin supply becomes disconnected and infusion site infections may occur

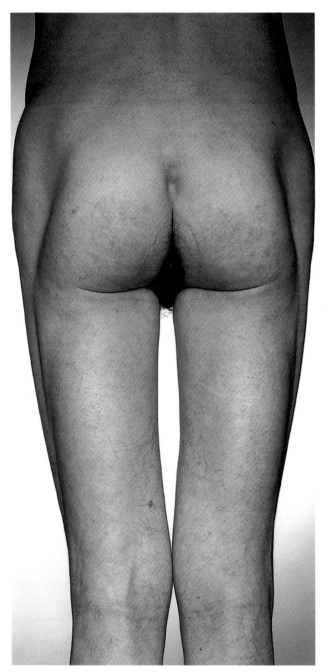

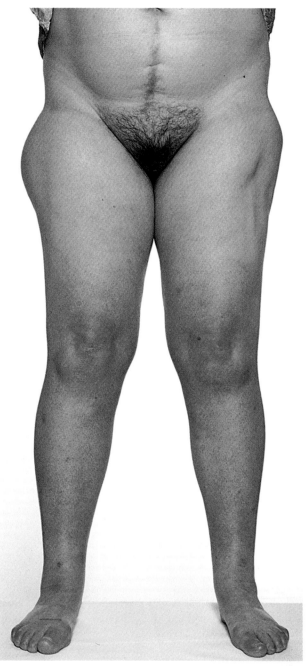

Figure 63 Insulin lipoatrophy manifests as depressed areas of skin owing to underlying fat atrophy. This was common before the advent of purified porcine and, more especially, human insulin. Several rare syndromes of lipoatrophy associated with diabetes have been described, and are characterized by insulin-resistant diabetes and absence of subcutaneous adipose tissue, either generalized or partial. These syndromes constitute a heterogeneous group, some of which are congenital and others of which are acquired

Figure 64 This patient has both insulin lipid hypertrophy and lipoatrophy. The lipid hypertrophy is seen in the lateral thigh and buttock regions where insulin has been injected. If the same injection site is used over many years, a soft fatty dermal nodule, often of considerable size, develops, possibly owing to the lipogenic action of insulin. Patients should be discouraged from using such sites as variation in insulin absorption may occur, leading to erratic control

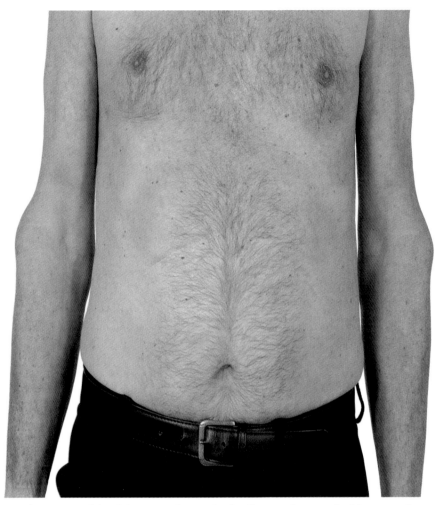

Figure 65 This patient has areas of lipid hypertrophy on both elbows. This is a highly unusual site to encounter lipid hypertrophy and a highly unusual site for insulin injection. His glycemic control, as a consequence, was very unstable but improved when he was persuaded to inject elsewhere on a rotational basis

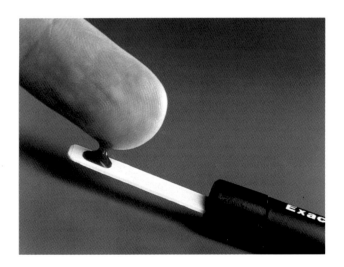

Figure 66 Blood glucose self-monitoring technique. A drop of blood is applied to a strip inserted into a pen meter. The drop of blood produces an electrical current proportional to its glucose concentration. No timing or wiping of the blood is necessary, although the timing sequence must be started by hand. Self-monitoring of blood glucose has become an integral part of modern insulin treatment. It allows patients to make their own adjustments to insulin dosages and helps to avoid hypoglycemia. Self-monitoring increases the patients' role in their own management and gives a greater sense of being in control of their condition. There is as yet no consensus on how often patients should check their blood glucose, and the role of self-monitoring in type 2 diabetes mellitus remains in dispute

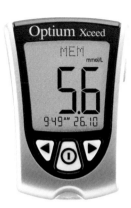

Figure 67 The Optium Xceed meter has the unique ability to measure both blood glucose and blood ketone levels. Not only are these functions useful in hospital patients with diabetic metabolic decompensation, but also they can be very helpful in allowing diabetic patients in the community to detect impending ketosis and thus take corrective action to prevent diabetic ketoacidosis

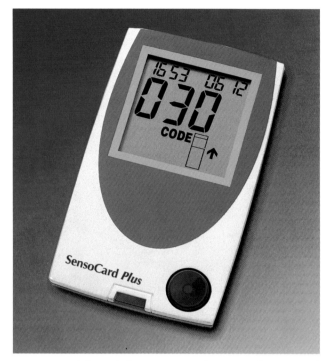

Figure 68 Many diabetic patients have significant visual loss due to diabetic retinopathy. Such loss makes conventional home blood glucose meters difficult to use. The newly developed SensoCard Plus meter is a novel talking blood glucose meter which uses biosensor technology to measure blood glucose and then produces the result using synthesized speech

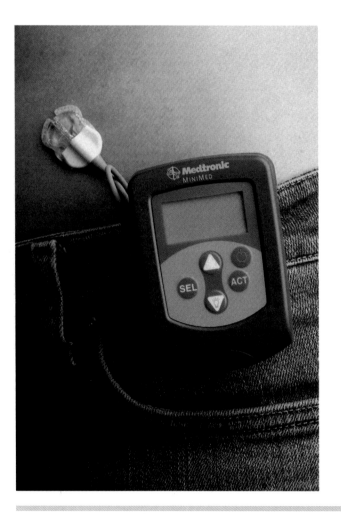

Figure 69 The MiniMed continuous glucose monitoring system is designed to monitor glucose levels in interstitial fluid, that are thought to be almost always comparable with blood glucose levels. A sensor is inserted under the skin of the anterior abdominal wall and interstitial glucose levels are sensed every 10 s and averaged over 5 min. Glucose sensors are worn for a maximum of 3 days and calibrated on the basis of four or more capillary glucose readings each day. Data are stored in the monitor and downloaded to an external computer and viewed in a graphical format

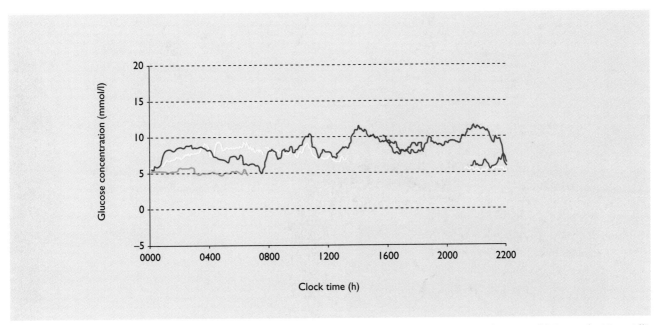

Figure 70   This profile shows very stable blood glucose control with most values between 5 and 10 mmol/l (90 and 180 mg/dl)

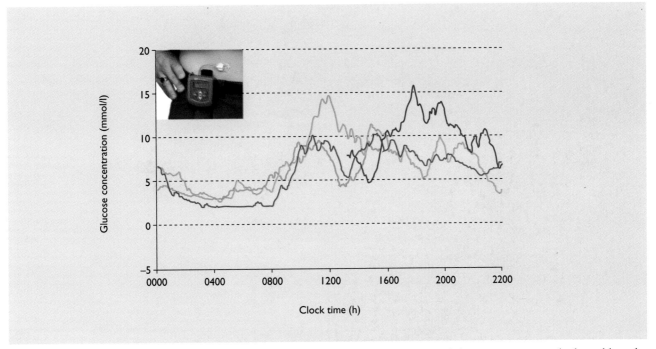

Figure 71   Data from continuous glucose monitoring may reveal surprising patterns of glucose excursions which could not be predicted from intermittent self blood glucose monitoring. These profiles show that the patient was frequently hypoglycemic during the night, while glucose control during the day was poor. Such information can lead to more focused adjustments of insulin regimens and improvement of overall glycemic load

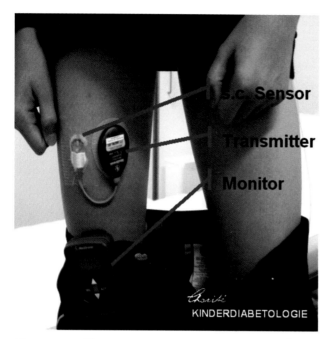

Figure 72 This patient is wearing a Guardian® RT, continuous real-time glucose monitor. The sensor measures interstitial fluid glucose levels providing up to 288 glucose readings per day. The glucose sensor is connected to a transmitter that communicates with a monitor using radiofrequency technology to display real-time glucose values every 5 minutes on the monitor screen. Alarm thresholds can be set to alert patients when glucose levels become too high or too low. Unfortunately, the device is prohibitively expensive as is the cost of the sensors

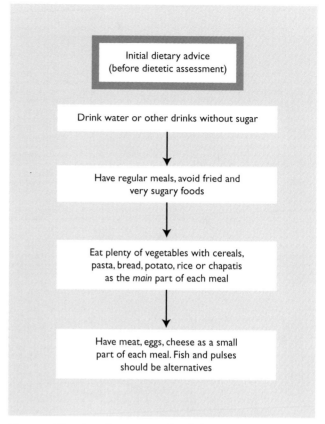

Figure 73 At diagnosis, all diabetic patients need immediate advice about what they should and should not eat. This may be given by the family physician, practice or specialist nurse, or hospital ward staff. It should be kept simple until a dietician can give more detailed recommendations (see Figure 74)

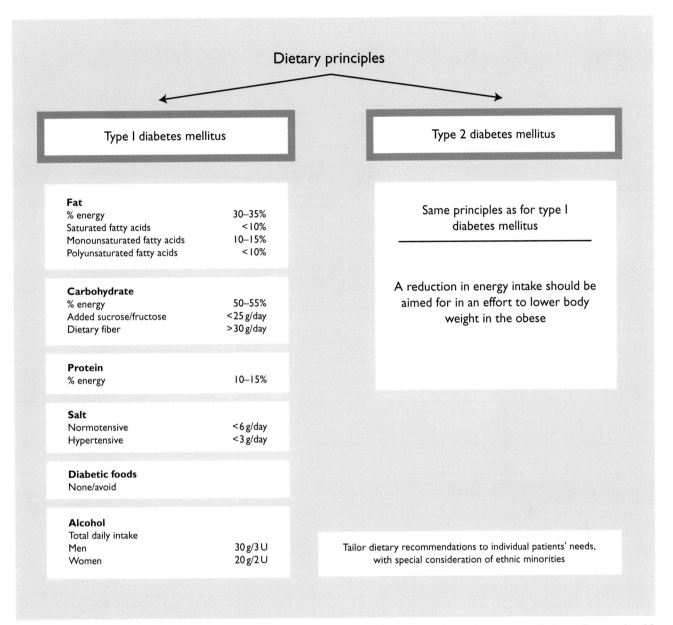

Dietary principles

Type 1 diabetes mellitus

Fat
% energy — 30–35%
Saturated fatty acids — <10%
Monounsaturated fatty acids — 10–15%
Polyunsaturated fatty acids — <10%

Carbohydrate
% energy — 50–55%
Added sucrose/fructose — <25 g/day
Dietary fiber — >30 g/day

Protein
% energy — 10–15%

Salt
Normotensive — <6 g/day
Hypertensive — <3 g/day

Diabetic foods
None/avoid

Alcohol
Total daily intake
Men — 30 g/3 U
Women — 20 g/2 U

Type 2 diabetes mellitus

Same principles as for type 1 diabetes mellitus

A reduction in energy intake should be aimed for in an effort to lower body weight in the obese

Tailor dietary recommendations to individual patients' needs, with special consideration of ethnic minorities

Figure 74 The importance of diet in the treatment of diabetes cannot be overemphasized. Patients and their relatives should have open access to consultation with a professional dietician. The dietary principles recommended do not differ greatly from the national recommendations for the general population

	Dose range	Dose distribution	Half-life
Sulfonylureas			
Tolbutamide	1.5–2.0 g	Divided	3–8 h
Chlorpropamide	100–500 mg	Single	35 h
Glibenclamide	2.5–20 mg	Single or divided	5 h
Glibornuride	12.5–75 mg	Single or divided	8 h
Glipizide	2.5–20 mg	Single or divided	4 h
Gliclazide	40–320 mg	Single or divided	12 h
Gliquidone	15–180 mg	Single or divided	4 h
Glimepiride	1–6 mg	Single	5–8 h
Meglitinides			
Repaglinide	0.1–16 mg	Divided	1 h
Nateglinide	60–540 mg	Divided	1.5 h
Biguanides			
Metformin	1.0–3.0 g	Divided	1.5–4.5 h
α-Glucosidase inhibitors			
Acarbose	50–600 mg	Single or divided	N/A
Miglitol	50–300 mg	Single or divided	N/A
Thiazolidinediones (glitazones)			
Rosiglitazone	4–8 mg	Single or divided	3–4 h
Pioglitazone	15–45 mg	Single	5–6 h

Figure 75 Many drugs are marketed for the treatment of type 2 diabetes, but most centers confine themselves to the use of one sulfonylurea, metformin and the glitazones with more sporadic use of acarbose and the meglitinides. The United Kingdom Prospective Diabetes Study has testified to the benefit of the use of metformin alone in obese patients and confirmed the safety of sulfonylureas. The PROactive study (PROspective pioglitAzone Clinical Trial in macro Vascular Events) of the use of pioglitazone in patients with type 2 diabetes and evidence of established macrovascular disease showed a lower proportion of patients reaching the secondary composite end points of all-cause mortality, non-fatal myocardial infarction and stroke with no effect on the more extensive primary end points. In most countries the meglitinides and α-glucosidase inhibitors are being used less frequently. Avandamet is a useful combination drug containing rosiglitazone and metformin. Glucophage SR, a slow-release version of metformin, may be given once daily and may have fewer gastrointestinal side-effects

4 Treatment of children and adolescents with diabetes

The importance of effective strategies for the treatment of diabetes in children and adolescents is accentuated by the knowledge that time-trend data, for countries where it is available, have demonstrated a clear increase in incidence of type 1 diabetes mellitus (DM) in these age groups. Such an increase suggests changes in environmental factors with the larger increase in children < 5 years of age suggestive of factors operative in early life. As alluded to elsewhere, cases of type 2 DM related to obesity are now being encountered, especially in high-risk ethnic groups.

Treatment strategies must incorporate knowledge of developmental milestones and behavioral, physiologic, psychologic and social factors that operate in this age group and impact so strongly on any chronic disease management program in children. Emotional problems are common, but controversy exists as to whether these have any long-term sequelae. Some studies have suggested that the onset of diabetes is associated with adjustment disorders which seemed to confer an increased risk of psychiatric problems later in life. A recent prospective study of adolescents with type 1 DM from Australia has documented the exhibition of a broad range of psychiatric diagnoses 10 years after disease onset, with females and adolescents with pre-existing psychologic problems being at particular risk.

Great skill by experienced teams comprising pediatric diabetic specialist nurses, dieticians, pediatric endocrinologists and child psychologists is needed to coordinate the effort to help diabetic children and their parents manage the diabetic condition. Difficult behavioral problems do occur in some children including denial of the disease, manipulative behavior and deliberate insulin overdosage and insulin omission. Frequent admissions with hypoglycemia or ketoacidosis usually reflect underlying emotional conflict. Such problems require a very sensitive approach to their management.

Most children (and their parents) rapidly become confident with insulin injections and self blood glucose monitoring. Older children (aged 8–12 years) are encouraged to self-inject. Childhood lasts a long time and, in order to minimize the risk of onset of microvascular complications, an attempt to achieve reasonable glycemic control should be made. This is often not easy to attain especially during puberty when glycemic control deteriorates. In a comparison of metabolic control in nearly 3000 children and adolescents with type 1 DM in 18 countries, the mean HbA$_{1c}$ was 8.6% with wide variation between centers. The degree of control achieved depends, to a certain extent, on many of the factors discussed above and often a compromise involving the child, the parents and the diabetologist has to be arrived at. Authoritarian approaches, especially during puberty, are likely to fail.

Total daily insulin requirements in children with type 1 DM are around 0.8 units/kg/24 h, increasing to 1.0–1.5 units/kg/24 h in mid-puberty. The principles of insulin therapy in children are broadly similar to those in adults. For reasons of simplicity or practicability, in many countries the standard insulin regimen consists of a twice-daily injection of a mixture of short-acting and isophane insulins either free-mixed into a syringe or, increasingly commonly, as a fixed mixture using a pen device. Two-thirds of the total daily dose is usually given at breakfast and one-third with the evening meal. A three-injection regimen, where the evening injection is split into a rapidly acting injection before the evening meal followed by an isophane injection before bed, is favored in some countries. More recently, newer preparations of more rapidly acting insulin analogs (lispro or aspart) with their protamine retarded counterparts (e.g. lispro/neutral protamine lispro, (Humalog Mix25®) aspart/neutral protamine aspart, NovoMix 30®) have become very popular and have certain advantages in children as they can be injected immediately before or even shortly after eating, the latter mode of administration allowing adjustment of the dose given according to the amount of food ingested (or refused).

Towards puberty and early adulthood, a greater need for flexibility emerges and, as the child becomes more independent, encouragement should be given to move towards multiple injection therapy with three injections of soluble or analog insulin with meals and twice-daily injections of isophane or a night-time dose of isophane insulin. Long-acting insulin analogs – insulin glargine and insulin detemir – are widely used in adults and are likely to prove useful in the treatment of adolescents particularly with regard to the prevention of nocturnal hypoglycemia. As in adults a typical regimen would be an insulin analog injected three times daily at meal times with long-acting analog injected once daily to provide a basal insulin supply usually before bed or at breakfast. At present few data are available examining the use of detemir in the pediatric population.

In children, who have less subcutaneous fat, the needle should not penetrate more than 3–5 mm to avoid intramuscular administration. It may be better to inject rapidly acting insulins into the abdomen where absorption is faster and delayed-action insulins into the thigh where absorption is slower. Continuous subcutaneous insulin infusion (CSII) is a perfectly acceptable method of insulin administration and is increasingly used within the pediatric diabetic population and has been associated in adolescents with less reported hypoglycemia, sustained improvements in HbA_{1c} after 12 months and a lower total daily insulin dose.

BIBLIOGRAPHY

Mortensen HB, Hougaard P. Comparison of metabolic control in a cross-sectional study of 2873 children and adolescents with IDDM from 18 countries. The Hvidore Study Group on Childhood Diabetes. Diabetes Care 1997; 20: 714–20

Northam EA, Matthews LK, Anderson PJ, et al. Psychiatric morbidity and health outcome in type 1 diabetes – perspectives from a prospective longitudinal study. Diabet Med 2005; 22: 152–7

Williams RM, Dunger DB. Insulin treatment in children and adolescents. Acta Paediatr 2004; 93: 440–6

5   Diabetes and surgery

It is well recognized, by both patients themselves and their usual advisors, that the treatment of diabetes in hospitalized diabetic patients is often suboptimal. A lack of knowledge of current treatment strategies and lack of familiarity with newer insulins, pen devices and newer hypoglycemic agents by ward staff contributes to substandard care, but can be overcome by the development, distribution and promotion of good treatment protocols, devised by the diabetic team to cover common situations. Many hospitals have now created in-patient diabetic specialist nurses to facilitate this with back-up from the diabetologist to help with more difficult or unusual cases. This is all the more important as many patients undergoing surgery will have diabetes and the metabolic stress of surgical procedures may lead to adverse outcomes if not properly managed. Diabetic patients undergoing surgery are at special risk of hyperglycemia and ketosis, hypoglycemia, perioperative complications such as wound infection, and iatrogenic problems of blood glucose control.

Factors to consider in the management of diabetic patients are the severity of surgical trauma and its duration, the pre-existing diabetes treatment and the extent of the patient's endogenous insulin reserves. Patients with type 1 diabetes and, for practical purposes, those with type 2 diabetes treated with insulin, are assumed to have no endogenous insulin and hence will require to be covered during surgery with exogenous insulin. Other patients will only require insulin therapy for major surgical procedures.

Protocols for the management of diabetes during surgery need to be simple, practicable, easily understood and, above all, safe. Avoidance of the pursuit of normoglycemia should be advised and it is perfectly acceptable to recommend a target range for blood glucose of around 6–10 mmol/l (108–180 mg/dl). Glucose levels much above this should be avoided as they may interfere with the wound healing process or be associated with increased postoperative infection rates.

Preoperative assessment is most important in diabetic patients undergoing surgery and close liaison between the anesthetist, surgeon and diabetes team is highly desirable, if not vital, in most cases. In general terms, although not always easy to achieve, all patients undergoing surgery who have diabetes should be operated on in the morning. The following treatment principles apply for type 2 patients not on insulin and for insulin-treated patients.

TYPE 2 DIABETES NOT ON INSULIN THERAPY

When pre-existing glycemic control is good and minor surgery only is planned, breakfast and oral agents are omitted on the morning of surgery (long-acting sulfonylureas should be omitted on the day prior to surgery). Dextrose infusions should be avoided and blood glucose checked every 2 hours. Postoperatively, oral agents may be recommended at the time of the next meal. When glycemic control is poor or major surgery is planned, it is desirable to admit the patient before the day of operation to optimize blood glucose control with short- or intermediate-acting insulins. On the day of surgery, breakfast is omitted and the surgery covered with intravenous insulin and glucose (see later). Postoperatively, subcutaneous insulin is continued until blood glucose levels are stable when the patient can restart oral therapy.

PATIENTS ON INSULIN THERAPY

Patients on insulin therapy having anything other than a minor surgical procedure should, optimally, be admitted prior to the day of planned surgery to allow stabilization of the blood glucose levels. On the day of surgery, which, as stated above, should always be in the morning, an intravenous infusion of insulin and glucose should be set up with potassium supplementation. Most centers utilize a continuous intravenous infusion of insulin via a pump driving a syringe containing 50 units of soluble insulin made up to 50 ml with normal saline, with the rate of insulin infusion being determined by the ambient hourly blood glucose level according to a preset protocol together with a separate infusion of 5% dextrose with added potassium through either a separate line or the insulin infusion being 'piggy-backed' into the dextrose infusion line.

An alternative regimen is the GKI (glucose–potassium–insulin) regimen whereby 15 units of soluble insulin with 10 mmol of potassium chloride is added to a 500 ml bag of 10% dextrose and the mixture is infused over 5 hours. If blood glucose levels are not controlled within the target range, then an appropriate alteration to the amount of insulin delivered must be effected by substituting a newly prepared bag with a different insulin dosage. Potassium supplements in both regimens may need to be altered according to measured plasma electrolytes.

The intravenous glucose, insulin, potassium regimen by whichever method is continued after the operation until the first postoperative meal when subcutaneous insulin is administered and the insulin infusion continued for a period that will depend on the time absorption profile of the insulin administered subcutaneously.

The above-mentioned protocols cover the broad generality of situations managed by the non-specialist. Specialist teams, with extensive experience of the management of perioperative diabetes, may modify them according to circumstances at the time.

6 Acute complications of diabetes

HYPOGLYCEMIA

Hypoglycemia is the greatest fear of patients treated with insulin. Hypoglycemia in patients with type 1 diabetes is a major source of disruption to their lives. It also occurs in patients treated with sulfonylureas, although to a lesser extent. Over 30% of insulin-treated diabetic patients experience hypoglycemic coma at least once in their lives, and approximately 3% experience frequent and severe episodes. In the Diabetes Control and Complications Trial, the incidence of severe hypoglycemia was much greater and was approximately three times higher in the intensively treated group. Severe hypoglycemia occurred more often during sleep. The main causes are excessive doses of insulin or sulfonylureas, inadequate or delayed ingestion of food and sudden or prolonged exercise, although such factors caused only a minority of episodes of severe hypoglycemia in the trial.

Death from hypoglycemia is rare and often is associated with the excessive use of alcohol or with deliberate insulin overdose. Unexpected deaths, thought to be attributable to hypoglycemia, are reported in young people with type 1 diabetes who are usually found dead in bed. Such deaths may be caused by hypoglycemia-induced cardiac dysrhythmia, although this remains unproven.

Acute hypoglycemia produces autonomic symptoms (such as sweating, tremor, palpitations and hunger) or neuroglycopenic symptoms (impaired cognitive function, such as difficulty in concentrating and incoordination). If neuroglycopenic symptoms occur without prior warning of autonomic symptoms, unconsciousness may develop.

Mild hypoglycemia responds quickly to glucose ingestion, but semiconscious or unconscious patients require intravenous dextrose (30 ml of a 20% solution) followed by oral glucose on recovery of consciousness. Intramuscular glucagon (1 mg), which stimulates hepatic glycogenolysis, is also a useful measure and can be given by a friend or relative.

In semiconscious patients, a 40% glucose gel (Glucogel®, formerly Hypostop, BBI Healthcare) can be smeared inside the cheeks and massaged to produce mucosal absorption of glucose. Failure to recover consciousness after intravenous glucose may be associated with cerebral edema and has a poor prognosis. Patients may respond to intravenous steroids or to mannitol.

Patients experiencing recurrent hypoglycemia need to liaise with their medical or specialist nursing advisors to determine the cause and to establish appropriate measures of prevention. When patients experience hypoglycemic unawareness, a strategy of loosening blood glucose control with strict avoidance of low blood glucose levels (< 4 mmol/l; 70 mg/dl) is advised and has been shown to be associated with a resumption of awareness of hypoglycemia.

Recurrent hypoglycemia and hypoglycemic unawareness pose particular problems for drivers and for those engaged in certain high-risk occupations, e.g. operating heavy machinery. Patients should be advised strictly to avoid such activities until these problems can be eliminated with the help of the diabetic team.

DIABETIC KETOACIDOSIS AND HYPEROSMOLAR NON-KETOACIDOTIC COMA

Diabetic ketoacidosis is the main cause of death in type 1 diabetic patients under 20 years of age. Its cardinal features are hyperketonemia, metabolic acidosis and hyperglycemia. Although diabetic ketoacidosis may occur at any age, it is most commonly seen in younger patients. It is often precipitated by infection and, more rarely, by another concurrent illness, such as myocardial infarction. Many cases occur in newly identified type 1 diabetic patients. Occasionally, it is precipitated by the deliberate omission of insulin injections. In many instances, no identifiable cause is found. Infection is the most common precipitating cause with new cases of diabetes being the second most common. Some patients have frequent recurrent episodes of ketoacidosis of no identifiable cause – they are usually females under 20 years of age. Deliberate omission or under-dosage of insulin is probably the cause in such patients. Ketoacidosis can occur in patients with type 2 diabetes as a consequence of severe infections and other intercurrent illness.

Diabetic ketoacidosis is characterized clinically by symptoms of nausea, vomiting, thirst, polyuria and, occasionally, abdominal pain accompanied by signs of dehydration, acidotic respiration, ketones on the breath, hypothermia and altered consciousness. Detailed biochemical assessment and monitoring (of urea, electrolytes, glucose and arterial gases) are mandatory in the management of this condition and a search should be undertaken for the underlying cause (by chest radiography or urine and blood cultures, for example). If a treatable underlying cause is found it should be treated promptly.

Successful treatment necessitates vigorous fluid replacement, correction of potassium deficiency, continuous intravenous insulin infusion, attention to acid–base status and treatment of the underlying cause where identifiable. Fluid replacement is with isotonic saline until the blood glucose falls below about 14 mmol/l (250 mg/dl), when 5% dextrose is substituted and infused at a rate of approximately 250 ml/h. Severe hypernatremia (plasma sodium > 155 mmol/l) or marked plasma hyperosmolality (> 350 mosm/kg) may require the use of hypotonic, rather than isotonic,

saline on a short-term basis. Approximately 6–10 liters of fluid may be required during the first 24 h, with 1 liter of saline being infused every hour for the first 2–3 h. Soluble insulin (Human Actrapid, Novo Nordisk or Humulin S, Eli Lilly) is given by continuous intravenous infusion usually at an initial rate of 5–10 units/h to produce steady plasma insulin concentrations to inhibit lipolysis and hence ketogenesis, to inhibit hepatic glucose production and to enhance disposal of glucose and ketone bodies by peripheral tissues. Hourly capillary blood glucose levels are checked to adjust the insulin infusion rate to maintain the blood glucose concentration between 5 and 10 mmol/l (90 and 180 mg/dl). The role of bicarbonate administration in diabetic ketoacidosis is controversial and unproven, but many advocate its use in severe acidosis with blood pH levels < 7.0.

Despite these and other measures, the overall mortality from diabetic ketoacidosis is around 7%. Cerebral edema, a rare and poorly understood cause of death in diabetic ketoacidosis, may respond to intravenous mannitol or dexamethasone. Hyperosmolar non-ketoacidotic coma carries an even greater mortality of around 30% of cases and is characterized by the insidious development of severe hyperglycemia, with resultant dehydration, and prerenal uremia unaccompanied by ketoacidosis.

Hyperosmolar non-ketoacidotic coma usually affects the middle-aged or elderly who have undiagnosed type 2 diabetes. Precipitating factors include infection, diuretic therapy and ingestion of glucose-rich drinks. Coma is more common in this condition than in diabetic ketoacidosis. Fluid, electrolyte and insulin replacement should be similar to that recommended for the treatment of diabetic ketoacidosis. In addition, there is an increased risk of thromboembolic disease with this condition. Prophylactic low-dose heparin (5000 units subcutaneously every 8 h) is often recommended if patients are immobile, have established thromboembolic disease or have other risk factors. Low molecular weight heparin by once-daily subcutaneous injection is easier to administer. However, the role of routine prophylactic anticoagulation in diabetic hyperglycemic emergencies remains unclear and many advocate anticoagulation with heparin only when there is definite evidence of thromboembolic disease.

BIBLIOGRAPHY

Cryer PE, Fisher JN, Shamoon H. Hypoglycemia. Diabetes Care 1994; 17: 734–55

Frier BM, Fisher BM, eds. Hypoglycemia and Diabetes. London: Edward Arnold, 1993

Kitabchi AE, Umpierrez GE, Murphy MB, et al. Management of hyperglycaemic crises in patients with diabetes. Diabetes Care 2001; 24: 131–53

Schade DS, Eaton RP, Alberti KGGM, Johnston DG. Diabetic Coma, Ketoacidotic and Hyperosmolar. Albuquerque: University of New Mexico Press, 1981

Small M, Alzaid A, MacCuish AC. Diabetic hyperosmolar non-ketoacidotic decompensation. Q J Med 1988; 66: 251–7

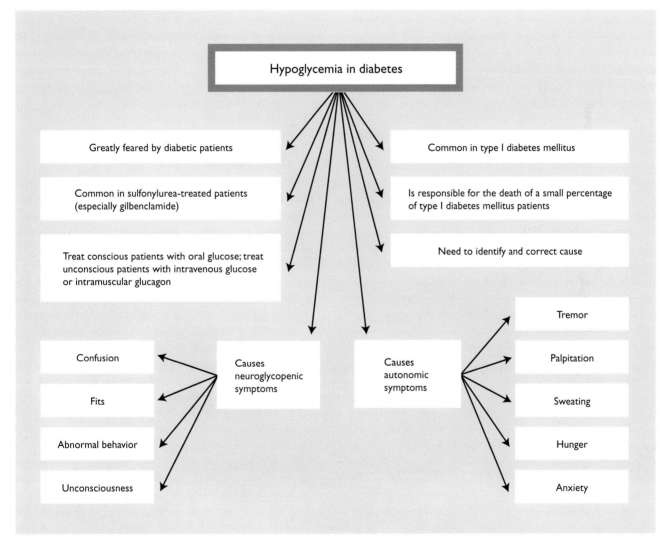

Figure 76 Hypoglycemia is a major problem for insulin-treated diabetic patients; over 30% of such patients experience hypoglycemic coma at least once. Around 10% experience coma in any given year and around 3% are incapacitated by frequent severe episodes. Hypoglycemia is usually due to an excessive dose of insulin, reduced or delayed ingestion of food, or increased energy expenditure owing to exercise. Identification of the cause, and appropriate remedial action and education, are mandatory. Patients treated with sulfonylureas frequently experience hypoglycemia

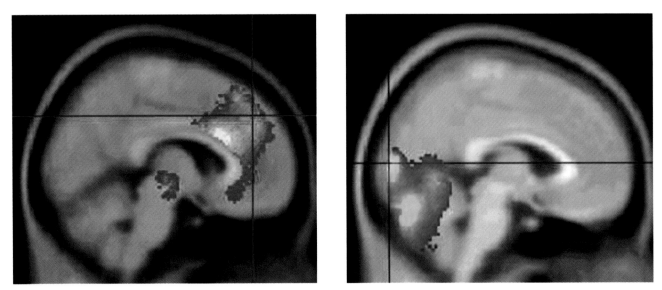

Figure 77 Hypoglycemia is associated with regional brain activation. Here CMG positron emission tomography (PET) has been used to measure changes in global and regional brain glucose metabolism. Hypoglycemia has been shown to be associated with activation of the brain stem, prefrontal cortex and anterior cingulate (yellow/orange indicates regions of increased glucose uptake and metabolism) and with reduced neuronal activation in the midline occipital cortex and cerebellar vermis (blue)

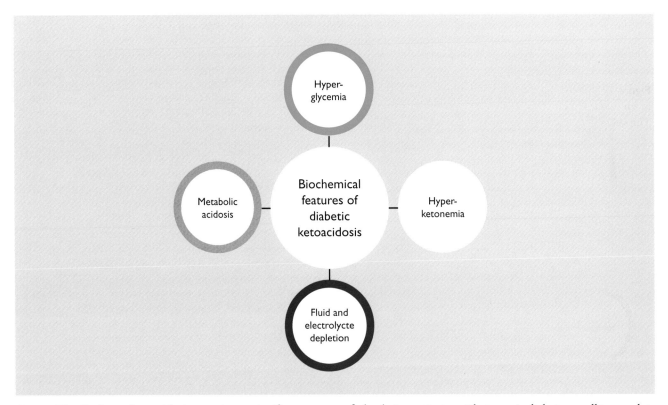

Figure 78 Diabetic ketoacidosis remains a significant cause of death in patients with type 1 diabetes mellitus and is characterized by marked hyperglycemia, hyperketonemia (usually detected by the presence of ketonuria), a low arterial pH, and fluid and electrolyte depletion with prerenal uremia. Treatment involves rehydration with saline, low-dose intravenous insulin infusion, potassium replacement, bicarbonate if arterial pH is < 7.0 and therapy directed at the underlying cause, if apparent

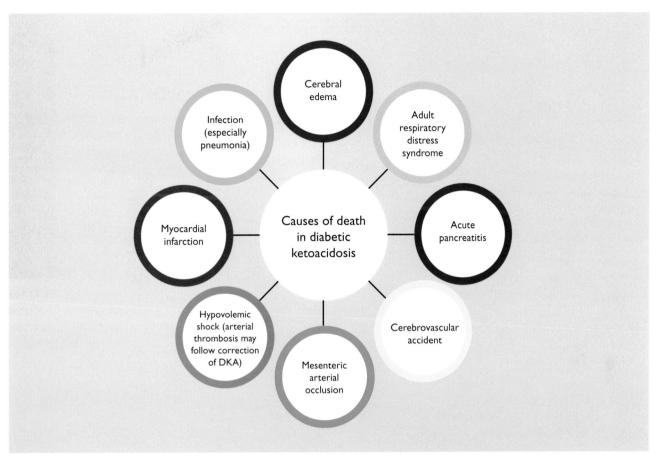

Figure 79 Myocardial infarction and infection are the most common causes of death in diabetic ketoacidosis. Cerebral edema is an uncommon and poorly understood cause of death, and appears to have a predilection for younger patients. Thromboembolic complications are an important cause of mortality. DKA, diabetic ketoacidosis

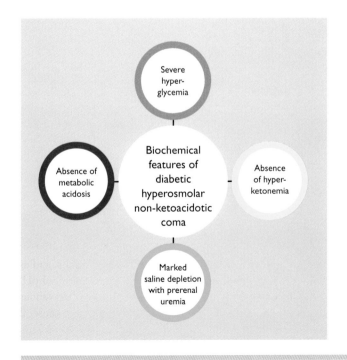

Figure 80 Hyperosmolar non-ketoacidotic coma usually affects middle-aged or elderly patients with previously undiagnosed type 2 diabetes mellitus. It is characterized by marked hyperglycemia (usually > 50 mmol/l; 900 mg/dl) and prerenal uremia without significant hyperketonemia and acidosis. Treatment is by fluid replacement, attention to electrolyte balance and insulin therapy as for diabetic ketoacidosis, and most patients will not ultimately require permanent insulin therapy. The condition has a high mortality owing to a high incidence of serious associated disorders and complications

7   Chronic complications of diabetes

The results of the Diabetes Control and Complications Trial in the USA have established unequivocally the relationship between glycemic control and the incidence or progression of diabetic microvascular complications. Such complications occur in both type 1 and type 2 diabetic patients, although the latter patients often die because of major vascular disease before microvascular complications become advanced. More than 40% of type 1 diabetic patients will survive for more than 40 years, half of them without developing significant microvascular complications. The United Kingdom Prospective Diabetes Study (UKPDS) has also provided pivotal information on the relationship between glucose control and complications in type 2 diabetes diabetes mellitus (DM). It has demonstrated, in a significant way, the beneficial effect of an improvement in blood glucose control on subsequent risk of developing specific diabetic complications.

DIABETIC RETINOPATHY

Both the incidence and prevalence of diabetic retinopathy are highest in type 1 diabetic patients with an early age of onset of diabetes. However, type 1 diabetic patients do not exhibit retinopathy at presentation, and the likelihood of developing significant diabetic eye disease in the first 5 years of the disease is small.

In contrast, type 2 diabetic patients may have retinopathy at presentation, presumably because they have had previously unrecognized type 2 diabetes for many years. The prevalence of retinopathy increases with the duration of diabetes. In general, significant visual impairment is usually caused by proliferative retinopathy in type 1 diabetes and by maculopathy in type 2 diabetes.

Background diabetic retinopathy is characterized by capillary dilatation and occlusion, microaneurysms, 'blot' hemorrhages and hard exudates (which are true exudates of lipid-rich material from abnormal vessels). This picture represents non-proliferative retinopathy and is not associated with visual loss unless hard exudates become extensive and involve the fovea. Preproliferative lesions, a harbinger of impending new vessel formation, include cottonwool spots, venous loops and beading, arterial narrowing and occlusion, and intraretinal microvascular abnormalities. The latter consist of abnormal dilated capillaries which are often leaky.

The importance of the recognition of preproliferative retinopathy is that it indicates the need for urgent referral to an ophthalmologist. New vessels originate from a major vein (occasionally from arteries) and appear in the retinal periphery or on the optic disc. They are much less common in type 2 diabetes than in type 1 diabetes. New vessels have a devastating impact on vision when they burst and produce sudden pre-retinal or vitreous hemorrhage. Contraction of associated fibroglial tissue may result in retinal detachment with resultant loss of vision, which may be profound if it affects the macula.

Diabetic maculopathy is the most common cause of visual loss in type 2 diabetes and may be exudative, edematous or ischemic. If left untreated, preproliferative retinopathy, proliferative retinopathy and maculopathy will all have an appalling prognosis for the patient's eyesight. All diabetic patients should be regularly screened for such changes and referred, where appropriate, for specialized ophthalmic assessment.

Laser photocoagulation can be used to destroy isolated new vessels or to undertake panretinal photocoagulation in cases of more severe proliferative retinopathy. The aim of the panretinal approach is to reduce retinal ischemia overall, thereby reducing the stimulus to new vessel formation.

Photocoagulation may also be used for the treatment of macular edema, with focal treatment given for discrete lesions and diffuse treatment for widespread capillary leakage and non-perfusion. Vitreoretinal surgery may be performed to treat severe vitreous hemorrhage and retinal detachment.

Detection of diabetic retinopathy at an early stage is essential. All diabetic patients should have regular ophthalmic examination. Screening programs for retinopathy should be designed to include all patients with diabetes in an attempt to avoid visual loss. The combination of direct ophthalmoscopy and digital retinal photography with measurement of visual acuity is often used. Suitably qualified optometrists have also been used in some screening programs.

DIABETIC NEPHROPATHY

Diabetic nephropathy is characterized by proteinuria, decreasing glomerular filtration rate and increasing blood pressure. In the absence of urinary infection or other renal disease, proteinuria in the order of >0.5 g/day is an indication of established diabetic nephropathy.

This degree of proteinuria is detectable by dipstick urine testing. However, it is recognized that this stage is preceded by a long phase of incipient nephropathy associated with microalbuminuria (30–300 mg/day) that is not detectable on dipstick testing. As microalbuminuria presages diabetic nephropathy, it allows the possibility of interventional treatment to slow the rate of progression of nephropathy.

Histologically, the diabetic kidney is characterized by increased glomerular volume secondary to basement membrane thickening and mesangial enlargement, hyaline deposits and glomerular sclerosis due to mesangial expansion and/or ischemia. Nephropathy is commonly seen in type 1 diabetic patients, especially in those who develop diabetes before the age of 15 years. Around 35% of type 1 diabetic patients will develop nephropathy; the incidence of new cases of nephropathy declines after approximately 16 years of diabetes. However, because type 2 diabetes is much more common, the majority of diabetic patients proceeding to end-stage renal failure have this form of diabetes.

The hypertension of diabetic nephropathy appears to be of renal origin and to occur after the onset of microalbuminuria. As proteinuria also reflects widespread vascular damage affecting both small and large vessels, the condition is associated with a poor prognosis unless special strategies are adopted. The causes of death include not only end-stage renal failure, but also myocardial infarction, cardiac failure and cerebrovascular accidents. Type 2 diabetic patients with nephropathy are more likely to die because of major vascular disease than uremia.

Peripheral vascular disease, neuropathy and retinopathy (usually proliferative) are virtually universal in diabetic nephropathy. Indeed, if neuropathy and retinopathy are not present, an alternative cause of the proteinuria should be sought. The sudden development of nephrotic syndrome, a rapid decline in renal function, hematuria and short duration of type 1 diabetes also indicate the need to seek an alternative cause, with the use of renal biopsy if necessary. If there is a marked discrepancy in size between the kidneys on ultrasound scanning, investigations should be conducted to exclude renal artery stenosis which is common in diabetes especially in type 2 diabetes with other evidence of vascular disease. Angiotensin-converting enzyme (ACE) inhibitors should be avoided in this situation. Regular monitoring of glomerular filtration rate and plotting the inverse of serum creatinine against time will give an indication of the rate of progression of nephropathy; however, this may be slowed by vigorous treatment of the associated hypertension, preferably with ACE inhibitors, which have the additional benefit of reducing intraglomerular pressure.

There is evidence that establishing strict glycemic control and adopting a diet of moderate protein restriction may also retard the progression of established nephropathy. With declining renal function, insulin requirements fall and, as most sulfonylureas and metformin undergo renal excretion or metabolism, these compounds should not be used in patients with renal failure; in such cases, insulin treatment is preferable, although some agents, such as gliclazide, which are cleared predominantly through the liver may be relatively safe.

With aggressive treatment of hypertension and hyperlipidemia and improvement of glycemic control, the need for renal replacement therapy may be delayed for several years. However, late referral of diabetic patients with advanced diabetic nephropathy to a nephrologist should be avoided: referral should be instigated when serum creatinine levels start to rise and certainly before they reach 300 μmol/l. Renal physicians prefer to see such patients earlier rather than later. Although renal transplantation offers the best method of treatment in suitable patients, hemodialysis is indicated in patients unsuitable for transplantation, while awaiting transplantation or following graft failure. Dialysis may need to be started at lower creatinine levels than in non-diabetic patients because of a tendency to increased fluid retention and volume-dependent hypertension. Vascular access and arterio-venous fistulae failures are additional problems for diabetic patients, as is difficulty achieving blood glucose control during hemodialysis. However, the prognosis of diabetic patients receiving hemodialysis, although poorer than in non-diabetics, has improved dramatically over the past 20 years.

Long-term survival of diabetic patients with continuous ambulatory peritoneal dialysis (CAPD) is possible. Survival rates may be lower than in non-diabetic patients receiving CAPD. Advantages of CAPD include the facts that vascular access is not required and that good glycemic control may be achieved by the intraperitoneal route of insulin.

Renal transplantation is the treatment of choice for those < 65 years who are free of significant cardiovascular disease, cerebrovascular disease and significant sepsis, and for whom a suitable donor may be found. Survival rates for diabetic patients who receive grafts from living donors are now almost the same as for non-diabetic patients, while results of cadaver transplantation, although less favorable, have improved greatly. Histologic changes compatible with diabetic nephropathy can be detected in most transplanted kidneys. In today's era, many diabetic patients with end-stage renal failure who require a transplant receive both a kidney and a pancreas at the same time.

A major Finnish study of 20 005 patients with type 1 diabetes showed that during a follow-up of 35 years the overall incidence of end-stage renal failure was only 2.2% at 20 years and 7.8% at 30 years after diagnosis. The risk of end-stage renal failure was virtually zero for the first 15 years after diagnosis. These data suggest a greatly improved renal outlook for patients with type 1 diabetes, especially for the under 5s. Overall survival has also improved.

DIABETIC NEUROPATHY

Diabetic neuropathy is a heterogeneous disorder that encompasses a wide range of abnormalities affecting proximal and distal peripheral sensory and motor nerves as well as the autonomic nervous system.

Prevalence

The exact prevalence of diabetic neuropathy is unknown, partly because of difficulties with definition. Reported prevalence rates vary from 10 to 90% in diabetic patients. It is known, however, that the risk of developing neuropathy is directly linked to the duration of diabetes: after 20 years of diabetes, around 40% of patients will have neuropathy. In patients attending a diabetic clinic, 25% reported symptoms, 50% were found to have neuropathy using a simple clinical test and almost 90% tested positive with more sophisticated tests. Neuropathy may be present at the time of diagnosis of type 2 diabetes, but neurologic complications occur equally in type 1 and type 2 diabetes. Neuropathy may lead to a significant reduction in quality of life and is a major determinant of foot ulceration and amputation.

Pathogenesis

The pathogenesis of diabetic neuropathy is unknown, but there is no doubt that hyperglycemia is an important factor. Pathologic studies demonstrate axonal degeneration with segmental demyelination and remyelination. Narrowing of the vasa nervorum may also be contributory. Neurophysiologic studies show reduced motor and sensory nerve conduction velocities. Abnormalities of the polyol pathway have been invoked as a cause of diabetic neuropathy. In animals, elevated glucose levels in peripheral nerves lead to an increased activity of aldose reductase, with consequent increased concentrations of sorbitol and fructose accompanied by a decrease in the polyol myoinositol. This may lead to reduced membrane sodium–potassium–ATPase activity. It has been postulated that such changes may be reversed by the use of aldose reductase inhibitors. Although these agents have been shown clinically to improve neural conduction velocity, their role in the treatment of diabetic neuropathy remains to be elucidated. Non-enzymatic glycosylation of nerve proteins and ischemia may also be significant factors in the development of diabetic neuropathy.

Chronic insidious sensory neuropathy

Chronic insidious sensory neuropathy is the most frequently encountered neuropathy in diabetes with paraesthesiae, discomfort, pain, distal sensory loss, loss of vibration sense and reduced or absent tendon reflexes. This type of neuropathy is usually refractory to treatment.

Acute neuropathy

Acute painful neuropathy is relatively uncommon and usually occurs in the context of poor glycemic control (or a sudden improvement in glycemic control). Lower limb pain may be particularly severe, and accompanied by muscle weakness and wasting. Recovery usually occurs within a year with good control of the diabetes.

Diabetic mononeuropathy

Diabetic mononeuropathies, affecting single nerves or their roots, also occur. They are usually of rapid onset and severe in nature, although eventual recovery is the rule in most cases. Such features may point to an acute vascular event as causation rather than chronic metabolic disturbance. Such neuropathies occur mainly in older patients, usually male. When two or more nerve palsies occur within a short time frame, mononeuritis multiplex must be excluded. Truncal radiculopathies, almost exclusively affecting the arm, are also encountered and cranial nerve lesions are seen relatively frequently. Third nerve palsies occur most commonly, although fourth, sixth and seventh nerve lesions are also described.

Proximal motor neuropathy

Proximal motor neuropathy (femoral neuropathy or diabetic amyotrophy) is a particularly devastating neurologic complication of diabetes. It can be identified clinically by certain common features. It primarily affects the elderly and is of gradual or abrupt onset beginning with pain in the thighs and hips or buttocks. Weakness of the proximal muscles of the lower limbs follows. The condition begins unilaterally but often spreads bilaterally and is associated with weight loss and depression. Slow, sometimes incomplete, recovery usually occurs but may take several months or a year or more. Electrophysiologic evaluation reveals a lumbosacral plexopathy, and the condition is now thought to be secondary to a variety of causes that occur more frequently in diabetes, such as chronic inflammatory demyelinating polyneuropathy, monoclonal gammopathy and inflammatory vasculitis. If found to be immune mediated, resolution may be very prompt with immunotherapy. Mononeuropathies must be distinguished from entrapment syndromes. Common entrapment sites in diabetic patients involve median, ulnar, radial, femoral and lateral cutaneous nerves of the thigh. Carpal tunnel syndrome occurs twice as frequently in diabetic patients compared with the normal population.

Diabetic autonomic neuropathy

Damage to the autonomic nervous system, or autonomic neuropathy, is seen in diabetic patients, although the exact prevalence is unknown. Tests of autonomic nerve function often reveal abnormalities in patients with no symptoms of autonomic dysfunction. These tests include the heart rate response to the Valsalva maneuver, to deep breathing and to moving from the supine to the erect posture, and the blood pressure response to sustained handgrip and standing up. Cardiovascular tests are relatively simple to perform, but evaluating the autonomic control of other systems, such as the gastrointestinal tract and micturition, is much more complex.

There is a wide spectrum of autonomic symptoms, including male impotence, postural hypotension, nocturnal diarrhea, gustatory sweating, diminished or absent sweating in the feet and loss of awareness of acute hypoglycemia. Gastric atony with loss of diabetic control in insulin-treated subjects and bladder enlargement with defective micturition are also reported. Resting tachycardia is a common sign. Many studies have suggested that, once symptomatic autonomic neuropathy is present, the prognosis for the patient is poor.

Treatment of diabetic neuropathy

Various agents, other than simple analgesics, have been utilized to try to diminish the distressing discomfort associated with painful diabetic neuropathies. Tricyclic antidepressants, which have a central action that modifies pain perception, are widely used and beneficial. Carbamazepine has been used in diabetic neuropathy. Other anticonvulsants, such as gabapentin, phenytoin, lamotrigine, topiramate and pregabalin, are used in the treatment of painful neuropathy. Gabapentin and pregabalin are well tolerated and often efficacious, while topiramate, although being effective, may not be so well tolerated. Other drugs studied and used in the treatment of painful diabetic neuropathy include lignocaine, mexiletine and tramadol.

Non-pharmacologic therapies include nerve stimulation therapies and electrical spinal-cord stimulation. Tricyclic antidepressants may be viewed as the first drug of choice with gabapentin a recommended alternative. Despite pharmacologic treatment many patients continue to experience pain or discomfort and treatment may be considered successful in patients who experience a moderate decrease in pain or improved function. Depletion of axonal neuropeptide substance P with capsaicin extracted from chilli peppers may help in some patients with C-fiber pain.

MAJOR VASCULAR DISEASE

Although microvascular disease is a major concern in diabetic patients, it should be emphasized that most patients with long-term type 1 DM and most patients with type 2 DM will die because of cardiovascular disease. Diabetic patients, particularly females, have an excess mortality owing to coronary artery disease compared with the non-diabetic control population. There is also an increased mortality due to peripheral vascular disease. Diabetic patients account for around 50% of all lower-limb amputations. Atheromatous lesions in diabetic patients are histologically identical to those in the non-diabetic population, but are more severe and widespread. Coronary artery disease may progress more quickly and hence present at a younger age. Although thrombolysis is effective, diabetic patients have a higher acute and delayed mortality after acute myocardial infarction mostly as a result of left ventricular failure. The Diabetes Mellitus Insulin GLucose infusion in Acute Myocardial Infarction (DIGAMI) study has suggested that the use of a glucose–insulin infusion and subsequent insulin treatment may significantly reduce 1-year mortality. Diabetes may also cause a specific cardiomyopathy in the absence of coronary artery disease.

Although risk factors for microvascular disease that pertain to the general population are also relevant to diabetic patients, hemostatic abnormalities (for example, decreased fibrinolysis or increased fibrinogen levels), hypertension and hyperlipidemia are particularly important in the latter. There is continuing debate over the atherogenic role of hyperinsulinemia and its relationship to the elevated levels of plasminogen activator inhibitor type 1 (PAI-1) described in diabetes.

HYPERTENSION

It is now abundantly clear that hypertension is a major risk factor in the development of diabetic complications, both macrovascular and microvascular. Therefore its detection and treatment are of vital importance in overall diabetic management. Hypertension is common in diabetes: it affects 10–30% of white patients with type 1 diabetes and 30–50% of those with type 2 diabetes. It is a major risk factor for stroke and coronary artery disease, but also aggravates nephropathy and retinopathy. Blood pressure starts to rise when microalbuminuria develops, and the close link between hypertension and nephropathy may be explained by genetic factors leading to an increased susceptibility to develop both associated with increased sodium–lithium counter-transport activity in red blood cells. It is now postulated that the common link between obesity, diabetes, hyperlipidemia and hypertension in type 2 diabetes is insulin resistance and associated hyperinsulinemia, either inherited or perhaps acquired through malnutrition in early life. Occasionally hypertension is associated with renal artery stenosis, and this should be investigated, and ACE inhibitors and angiotensin II receptor antagonists avoided, when this clinical suspicion arises.

Targets for blood pressure lowering should be lower than for the non-diabetic population because of the major adverse effect of hypertension in this group: a blood pressure of 130/80 should be aimed for and perhaps even lower in high-risk patients, e.g. those with nephropathy. The Blood Pressure Control Study incorporated into the UKPDS demonstrated that a tight blood pressure control policy achieving a mean blood pressure of 144/82 gave a reduced risk for any diabetes-related end point, diabetes-related deaths, stroke, microvascular disease, heart failure and progression of retinopathy. It also demonstrated that in many patients combination therapy was necessary to achieve this level of blood pressure control. However, effective blood pressure reduction is likely to be more achievable than effective blood glucose control.

ACE inhibitors are the first choice to treat diabetic hypertension, as not only are they effective but also they delay the progression of diabetic retinopathy and diabetic nephropathy (perhaps in the latter by reducing intraglomerular pressure). Such agents include captopril, enalapril, lisinopril, fosinopril and ramipril. The effect of ramipril in reducing the rates of death, myocardial infarction and stroke in a broad range of high-risk patients, about 40% of whom had diabetes, was demonstrated in the Heart Outcomes Prevention Evaluation Study (HOPE study) and is likely to extend to other drugs in this group.

When ACE inhibitors cannot be tolerated, e.g. owing to dry cough, then an angiotensin II receptor antagonist such as losartan, valsartan or irbesartan should be substituted. Beta-blockers are also helpful antihypertensive agents, especially post-myocardial infarct or when there is co-existing angina. They should be avoided in bronchial asthma or when there is severe peripheral vascular disease. Bendrofluazide at low dose (2.5 mg/day) effectively lowers pressure, but should be avoided in type 2 diabetes for fear of aggravating hyperglycemia. Indapamide may be a useful substitute. Calcium-channel blockers and α-receptor blockers, such as doxazosin are useful add-on drugs to achieve satisfactory blood pressure control.

THE DIABETIC FOOT

Foot ulcers are relatively common in patients with diabetes occurring in up to 15% of all diabetic patients.

The associated health-care costs are enormous. It has been estimated that the attributable cost for a patient's foot ulcer care is nearly $28 000 during the 2 years after diagnosis. Observational studies suggest that 6–43% of patients with a diabetic foot ulcer will ultimately progress to amputation. The costs associated with this are even more formidable. The tragedy is that such morbidity and costs result from lesions that may be prevented by the institution of, and compliance with, diabetic foot care policies.

The main causes of foot ulceration are neuropathy, medium and small vessel peripheral vascular disease and abnormal foot biomechanics. These factors are frequently compounded by bacterial infection with organisms such as *Staphylococcus aureus* and *Streptococcus pyogenes*, often accompanied by anaerobes such as *Bacteroides* species. Neuropathy is thought to be the main factor in over one-half of ulcers with trauma occurring as a result of loss of pain sensation. Minimal trauma, such as a foreign body in the shoes, ill-fitting shoes or walking barefoot on a hot surface may lead to devastating effects (see Figures 108 and 109). Excessive pressure loading on the sole, especially over the metatarsal heads and heels, predisposes to the formation of callus which can break down and lead to ulceration. Indeed callus is an important predictor of ulceration. Such excess pressure is generated by motor-nerve damage altering the posture of the foot, limited joint mobility and local deformities including Charcot arthropathy. Autonomic nerve damage leads to reduced sweating and a dry skin which may crack or split more easily allowing the ingress of infection. Atherosclerotic disease of the peripheral vessels, especially the small vessels, is common in diabetic patients and is a predisposing factor in most cases of diabetic foot ulceration. Ulcers attributable purely to ischemia are relatively rare and, as neuropathy usually co-exists, are described as neuro-ischemic as opposed to the more common neuropathic ulcers where neuropathy is the critical antecedent factor. When ulcers are infected they exhibit local signs of inflammation such as erythema, warmth and tenderness, although such signs might be unimpressive despite definite infection. Deep-seated infection and osteomyelitis are important to diagnose. If bone can be felt when probing an ulcer, osteomyelitis can be assumed. Deep infection is suggested by the presence of deep sinuses, a foul discharge and crepitus on palpating the foot.

It follows from the above discussion that risk factors for the development of diabetic foot ulcers include presence of neuropathy (and other microvascular complications), peripheral vascular disease, previous amputation and foot deformity together with previous foot ulceration, poor footcare advice and advanced age.

Management of diabetic foot ulceration is complicated and requires great expertise and experience, particularly because most, if not all, approaches to treatment are not evidence based. A multidisciplinary approach is warranted involving, as necessary, diabetologists, podiatrists, orthopedic surgeons, vascular surgeons, microbiologists, primary-care physicians, nurses and orthotists. Debridement and removal of slough and necrotic eschar is vital to promote healing. Surgical debridement may occasionally be necessary for an extensive lesion. Relief of pressure is a basic principle of management of all neuropathic ulcers using such methods as an insole encased in either a temporary shoe or plaster cast (total contact cast or Scotchcast boot). Dressings should be absorbent enough to deal with wound exudation. A moist wound environment may be preferable to encourage granulation tissue. Infection must be treated when present but may be difficult to determine as may be the causative organism. There is no consensus as to which antibiotic regimens to use. In the absence of deep infection, monotherapy with a broad-spectrum antibiotic, such as co-amoxiclav, is appropriate. Deep ulcers necessitate initial intravenous administration of a combination of antibiotics, such as ampicillin, flucloxacillin and metronidazole, changing to oral administration when the infection seems to be responding. Clindamycin is useful when there is a suspicion or proven osteomyelitis as it has good penetration into bone. Routine radiography may be helpful in showing the presence of gas or evidence of osteomyelitis. It often reveals calcification of the small vessels of the foot. Osteomyelitis can be confirmed by alternative imaging techniques such as magnetic resonance imaging (MRI) or white-cell scanning. In all cases a vascular assessment should be made and amputation may be necessary if there is extensive gangrene or spreading necrosis in a toxic patient. Revascularization may be possible for neuroischemic ulcers.

Many new and experimental treatments for diabetic foot ulcers have emerged in recent years. Dermagraft®, Smith and Nephew (cultured human dermis) and Apligraf®, Novartis (Graftskin) (bi-layered bioengineered skin substitute) have been shown to shorten healing time and to produce a significantly greater proportion of healed ulcers. Platelet-derived growth factor (becaplermin) has been used to heal small low-grade ulcers. Hyperbaric oxygen has been shown to accelerate the rate of healing and increase the number of wounds completely healed. Debridement with maggots is simple and effective for cleaning chronic wounds and initiating granulation. None of these techniques has become an accepted standard therapy for the treatment of diabetic foot ulcers and further assessments of efficacy and cost-effectiveness are required.

The assessment of foot ulcer risk, the dissemination of good foot care advice and early and urgent treatment of established ulceration are the mainstays of the prevention of amputation secondary to diabetic foot ulcers. Comprehensive screening programs and treatment programs have been shown to reduce the risk of amputation. Preventative podiatric care should be given to all patients at risk. Simple measures, such as the debridement of callus and the fitting of appropriate shoes, often with the help of an orthotist, may be all that is necessary to prevent one of the most devastating and feared complications of diabetes, amputation.

ERECTILE DYSFUNCTION IN DIABETES

In recent years, there has been a seismic change in the recognition and management of diabetic patients with erectile dysfunction (ED). Fundamental to this is the recognition that ED represents a vascular complication of the disease. Cardiovascular disease increases the risk of ED, but ED itself is probably a risk factor for cardiovascular disease. The estimated prevalence of ED in diabetic populations is of the order of 38–55% making it one of the most common complications of diabetes in men. ED in diabetes is most likely to be as a result of a defect in nitric oxide-mediated smooth-muscle relaxation as a consequence of autonomic nerve damage and endothelial dysfunction. Large vessel disease and hypertension may also contribute.

In today's climate, male diabetic patients with ED are much more likely to seek advice and treatment. Every opportunity for them to so do should be made available and routine enquiry into sexual function, especially in older patients, may well be appropriate. Few investigations are needed. Measuring serum testosterone might be helpful if sex drive is reduced. Other endocrine testing should only be undertaken in the rare situation when a clinical suspicion of hypogonadism exists. A detailed history should be taken to define the precise problem with sexual function.

If a diabetic male with ED wishes treatment for the condition, he should be offered an oral agent as first-line therapy assuming there is no contraindication. It is fruitless to try and determine whether the ED has a psychogenic component or not. Phosphodiesterase inhibitors, such as sildenafil (Viagra®), are the agents of choice. Inhibition of this enzyme diminishes the breakdown of nitric oxide via the second messenger cGMP. Sildenafil only works in the presence of sexual stimulation and has no effect on libido. It should be taken in a dose of 50–100 mg 1 hour before planned sexual activity and sexual activity may take place for about 4 hours after the 1 hour period. The commonest side-effects are headaches, dyspepsia and flushing. Sildenafil is not associated with an increased risk of cardiovascular events, although the resultant sexual activity may be. Treatment with nitrates is an absolute contraindication to the use of sildenafil as the combination may produce profound hypotension. Temporary visual changes have been reported. The success rate for sildenafil for the treatment of ED in diabetic men is about 60%.

Vardenafil and tadalafil are more recently introduced phosphodiesterase inhibitors. Vardenafil is a useful alternative to sildenafil and may be associated with a lower frequency of visual disturbance as a side-effect. It is worth trying when sildenafil has failed. Tadalafil has a much longer half-life than either sildenafil or vardenafil. The advantage of this is that is can be taken several hours before sexual activity rather than shortly beforehand. Additionally, its efficacy may persist for up to 36 hours after oral dosing.

Apomorphine, a centrally acting inducer of erections, is an alternative to phosphodiesterase inhibitors. Nausea is the main side-effect, however, this is much less frequent with the licensed sublingual preparation.

In those failing to respond to oral agents, erection may be induced by the intracavernosal injection of alprostadil (prostaglandin E). However, long-term discontinuation rates are high, penile pain is a relatively common side-effect of such therapy and patients must be warned of the much more serious complication of priapism which, if it occurs, necessitates urgent medical attention. An alternative mode of delivery of alprostadil is by the transurethral routine using a slender applicator to deposit a pellet containing alprostadil in polyethylene glycol. Such therapy, marketed as MUSE (Medicated Urethral System for Erection) has been successful in about 65% of diabetic men although often associated with penile pain. Long-term usage rates are not high and some men may actually prefer to inject intracavernosally.

Devices which produce a passive penile tumescence by applying a vacuum via a hand or battery operated pump are available. Penile engorgement is maintained using a rubber constriction ring at the base of the penis. Although rigidity sufficient for vaginal penetration may be induced in most patients, the quality of erection may not be as good as that achieved by pharmacologic methods and many couples may not find such a technique acceptable for a variety of reasons. For those who have failed to respond to the above approaches and with careful selection and counseling, the surgical implantation of a penile prosthesis can be a successful treatment for erectile failure.

NON-ALCOHOLIC STEATOHEPATOSIS

Non-alcoholic fatty liver disease, has recently become increasingly recognized and may progress to end-stage liver disease. It is histologically indistinguishable from the liver damage that is secondary to alcohol abuse, but occurs in people with no history of alcohol excess. Non-alcoholic fatty liver disease has a wide spectrum of liver damage ranging from simple steatosis to steatohepatitis, advanced fibrosis and cirrhosis. The combination of steatosis, infiltration by mononuclear or polymorphonuclear cells (or both), and hepatocyte ballooning and spotty necrosis is known as non-alcoholic steatohepatitis (NASH). Non-alcoholic fatty liver disease is the most common cause of abnormal liver blood results among adults in the USA. It is particularly common in those with combined diabetes and obesity: in a group of severely obese patients with diabetes, 100% were found to have mild steatosis, 50% had NASH and 19% had cirrhosis. Insulin resistance seems to be the most reproducible causative factor in the development of non-alcoholic fatty liver disease and NASH, and this condition is increasingly viewed as part of the spectrum of the metabolic syndrome.

Malaise and a sensation of fullness or discomfort in the right hypochondrium are recognized symptoms when symptoms exist and hepatomegaly is the only consistent physical sign. Mild to moderate elevation of liver enzymes is often the only laboratory abnormality and fatty infiltration of the liver produces a diffuse increase in echogenicity on ultrasonography as compared with the kidneys. Liver biopsy provides an ultimate diagnosis. No satisfactory drug therapy is available for this condition, but encouraging results have been obtained with gemfibrozil, metformin, ursodeoxycholic acid and glitazones.

THE SKIN IN DIABETES

A variety of disorders of the skin occur in patients with DM. Some of these conditions are associated with endocrine or metabolic disorders that may themselves cause diabetes.

Acanthosis nigricans

This skin manifestation is often missed on examination, but is, nevertheless, fairly frequently encountered in patients with DM especially in those with genetic syndromes of insulin resistance and the metabolic syndrome. It is characterized by a velvety, papillomatous, usually pigmented, overgrowth of the epidermis and occurs particularly in the axillae, neck, groin and inframammary areas (Figure 143). It may be caused by hyperinsulinemia induced stimulation of insulin-like growth factor (IGF)-1 receptors on keratinocytes.

Necrobiosis lipoidica diabeticorum

Necrobiosis is rare in patients with DM. Although traditionally thought of as a classical diabetic skin manifestation, it can also occur in patients without diabetes. Necrobiosis usually develops in young adults or in early middle life and is much more common in women than in men. The skin is the most commonly affected site and the appearance ranges from early dull red papules or plaques, through indurated plaques with skin atrophy often with telangiectactic vessels on a waxy yellowish background to actual skin ulceration (Figures 137 and 138). Treatment is controversial, largely unproven and usually ineffective. Intralesional

or topical corticosteroids or excision and skin grafting may have a limited role.

Diabetic dermopathy

These well circumscribed, atrophic, brownish scars commonly seen on the shin ('shin spots') occur in up to 50% of diabetic patients (Figure 140) and are also seen much less frequently in non-diabetic subjects. Although there is no effective treatment, they tend to regress over time.

Diabetic bullae

Tense blisters, more common in men than women, occurring most frequently on the lower legs and feet occur rarely in diabetic patients (Figure 142). They appear rapidly and heal after a few weeks.

Other

Other skin conditions encountered in diabetic patients are diabetic erythema, periungual telangiectasia, diabetic thick skin (linked with the formation of advanced glycation end-products), vitiligo (autoimmune destruction of melanocytes, Figure 136), eruptive xanthomata (caused by hypertriglyceridemia in diabetic dyslipidemia, Figures 148 and 149), migratory necrolytic erythema (associated with glucagonoma syndrome, Figure 141) and urticarial reactions to insulin allergy.

RARER MANIFESTATIONS OF DIABETES MELLITUS

Diabetic cheiroarthropathy

This rheumatic complication of diabetes manifests itself as limited joint mobility associated with thickening and tightening of the skin especially noticed on the dorsal surfaces of the hands. Resultant contraction prevents the affected patient from placing their hand flat on to a surface and from approximating the palmar surfaces of the hand – the 'prayer' hand sign (Figure 150). Although seen in both adult-onset type 1 and type 2 diabetes, it is most commonly encountered in children and young adults with type 1 DM often related to poor glycemic control and associated with other more specific diabetic complications such as retinopathy.

Dupuytren's contracture

Dupuytren's contracture (Figure 151) has a quoted prevalence varying between 20 and 63% in DM. Furthermore, in patients presenting with Dupuytren's contracture, a high prevalence of diabetes is found. It is more commonly found in elderly patients with a long duration of diabetes and may have an association with carpal tunnel syndrome.

Adhesive capsulitis of the shoulder

There are numerous reports of an association between periarthritis of the shoulder – 'frozen shoulder' – and DM and such patients are encountered frequently in routine diabetic follow-up clinics. This condition is characterized by pain and limitation of movement of the shoulder joint, both active and passive. Referral to a rheumatologist is appropriate.

BIBLIOGRAPHY

Aiello LP, Gardner TW, King GL, et al. Diabetic retinopathy. Diabetes Care 1998; 21: 143–56

Angulo P. Nonalcoholic fatty liver disease. N Engl J Med 2002; 346: 1221–31

Archer AG, Watkins PJ, Thomas PK, Sharma AK, Payan J. The natural history of acute painful diabetic neuropathy. J Neurol Neurosurg Psychiatr 1983; 46: 491–9

Arkkila PE, Kantola IM, Viikari JS, et al. Dupuytren's disease in type 1 diabetic patients: a five-year prospective study. Clin Exp Rheumatol 1996; 14: 59–65

Barnett AH, Dodson PM. Hypertension and Diabetes. London: Science Press Ltd, 1990

Bell DS. Diabetic cardiomyopathy. A unique entity or complication of coronary artery disease? Diabetes Care 1995; 18: 708–14

Bommer J. Attaining long-term survival when treating diabetic patients with ESRD by hemodialysis. Adv Ren Replace Ther 2001; 8: 13–21

British Multicentre Study Group. Photocoagulation for proliferative diabetic retinopathy: a randomised controlled clinical trial using the zenon arc. Diabetologia 1984; 26: 109–15

Chauhan A, Foote J, Petch MC, Schofield PM. Hyperinsulinemia, coronary artery disease and syndrome X. J Am Coll Cardiol 1994; 23: 364–8

Donnelly R, Emslie-Smith AM, Gardner ID, Morris AD. ABC of arterial and venous disease: vascular complications of diabetes. Br Med J 2000; 320: 1062–6

Drury PL. Hypertension. Baillières Clin Endocrinol Metab 1988; 2: 375–9

Dyck PJ, Thomas PK, Asbury AK, et al. Diabetic Neuropathy. Philadelphia: WB Saunders, 1987

Early Treatment of Diabetic Retinopathy Study Research Group. Photocoagulation for diabetic macular oedema. Arch Ophthalmol 1985; 103: 1796–806

Edmonds ME. The diabetic foot: pathophysiology and treatment. Clin Endocrinol Metab 1993; 15: 889–916

Eldor R, Raz I, Ben Yehuda A, Boulton AJM. New and experimental approaches to treatment of diabetic foot ulcers: a comprehensive review of emerging treatment strategies. Diabet Med 2004; 21: 1161–73

Estacio RO, Schrier RW. Diabetic nephropathy: pathogenesis, diagnosis, and prevention of progression. Adv Intern Med 2001; 46: 359–408

Ewing DJ, Campbell IW, Clarke BF. The natural history of diabetic autonomic neuropathy. Q J Med 1980; 193: 95–108

Ferris FL 3rd, Davis MD, Aiello LM. Treatment of diabetic retinopathy. N Engl J Med 1999; 341: 667–78

Finne P, Reunanen A, Stenman S, et al. Incidence of end-stage renal disease in patients with Type 1 diabetes. JAMA 2005; 294: 1782–7

Greene DA, Lattimer SA, Sima AAF. Sorbitol, phosphoinositides and sodium-potassium ATPase in the pathogenesis of diabetic complications. N Engl J Med 1987; 316: 599–606

Haffner SM. Epidemiology of insulin resistance and its relation to coronary artery disease. Am J Cardiol 1999; 84: 11J–14J

Ho T, Smiddy WE, Flynn HW Jr. Vitrectomy in the management of diabetic eye disease. Surv Ophthalmol 1993; 37: 190–202

Hutchinson A, McIntosh A, Peters J, et al. Effectiveness of screening and monitoring tests for diabetic retinopathy – a systematic review. Diabet Med 2000; 17: 495–506

Jacobson SH, Fryd D, Sutherland DER, Kjellstrand CM. Treatment of the diabetic patient with end-stage renal failure. Diabetes Metab Rev 1988; 4: 191–200

Jelinek JE. The skin in diabetes. Diabetic Med 1993; 10: 210–13

Kohner EM, Porta M, eds. Screening for Diabetic Retinopathy in Europe: A Field Guidebook. Copenhagen: WHO Regional Office for Europe, 1992

Kohner EM. Diabetic retinopathy. Br Med J 1993; 307: 1195–9

Lewis EJ, Hunsicker LG, Pain RP, Rohde RD. The effect of angiotensin-converting enzyme inhibition on diabetic nephropathy. N Engl J Med 1993; 329: 1456–65

Malmberg K. Prospective randomised study of intensive insulin treatment on long term survival after acute myocardial infarction in patients with diabetes mellitus. GIGAMI (Diabetes Mellitus, Insulin Glucose Infusion in Acute Myocardial Infarction) Study Group. Br Med J 1997; 314: 1512–15

McCulloch DK, Young RJ, Prescott RJ, Clarke BF. The natural history of impotence in diabetic men. Diabetologia 1984; 26: 437–40

Mead A, Burnett S, Davey C. Diabetic retinal screening in the UK. J R Soc Med 2001; 94: 127–9

Mogensen CE, ed. Microalbuminuria predicts clinical proteinuria and early mortality in maturity-onset diabetes. N Engl J Med 1984; 310: 356–60

Mogensen CE, ed. The Kidney and Hypertension in Diabetes Mellitus. Boston: Martinus Nijhoff Publishing, 1988

Mogensen CE, Cooper ME. Diabetic renal disease: from recent studies to improved clinical practice. Diabet Med 2004; 21: 4–17

Passadakis P, Oreopoulos D. Peritoneal dialysis in diabetic patients. Adv Ren Replace Ther 2001; 8: 22–41

Perez MI, Kohn SR. Cutaneous manifestations of diabetes mellitus. J Am Acad Dermatol 1994; 30: 519–31

Ramsey SD, Newton K, Blough D, et al. Incidence, outcomes, and cost of foot ulcers in patients with diabetes. Diabetes Care 1999; 22: 382–7

Reaven GM. Role of insulin resistance in human disease. Diabetes 1988; 37: 1595–607

Scobie IN, MacCuish AC, Barrie T, et al. Serious retinopathy in a diabetic clinic: prevalence and therapeutic implications. Lancet 1981; 2: 520–1

Shapiro LM. A prospective study of heart disease in diabetes mellitus. Q J Med 1984; 209: 55–68

Spruce MC, Potter J, Coppini DV. The pathogenesis of painful diabetic neuropathy: a review. Diabet Med 2003; 20: 88–98

Stern M. Natural history of macrovascular disease in type 2 diabetes. Role of insulin resistance. Diabetes Care 1999; 22 (Suppl 3): c2–5

Taylor KG, ed. Diabetes and the Heart. Tunbridge Wells: Castle House Publications, 1987

UK Prospective Diabetes Study Group. Tight blood pressure control and risk of macrovascular and microvascular complications in type 2 diabetes: UKPDS 38. Br Med J 1998; 317: 703–13

UK Prospective Diabetes Study Group. Efficacy of atenolol and captopril in reducing risk of macrovascular and microvascular complications in type 2 diabetes; UKPDS 39. Br Med J 1998; 317: 713–20

Vinik Al, Park TS, Stansberry KB, Pittenger GL. Diabetic neuropathies. Diabetologia 2000; 43: 957–73

Watkins PJ. The diabetic foot. Br Med J 2003; 326: 977–9

Young MJ, Boulton AJM, MacLeod AF, et al. A multicentre study of the prevalence of diabetic peripheral neuropathy in the United Kingdom hospital clinic population. Diabetologia 1993; 35: 150–4

Young RJ, Clarke BF. Pain relief in diabetic neuropathy: the effectiveness of imipramine and related drugs. Diabetic Med 1985; 2: 363–6

Young RJ, Ewing DJ, Clarke BF. Chronic remitting painful diabetic polyneuropathy. Diabetes Care 1988; 11: 34–40

Yusuf S, Sleight P, Pogue J, et al. Effects of an angiotensin-converting-enzyme inhibitor, ramipril, oncardiovascular events in high-risk patients. The Heart Outcomes Prevention Evaluation Study Investigators. N Engl J Med 2000; 342: 145–53

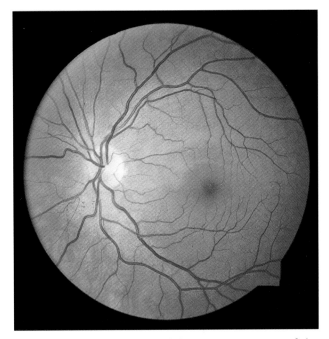

Figure 81 Normal fundus of the eye. Appreciation of the fundal abnormalities seen in diabetes must be based on a sound knowledge of the normal appearance

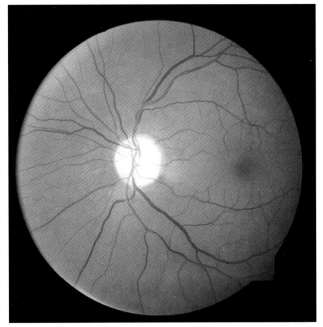

Figure 82 Optic atrophy in the DIDMOAD (diabetes insipidus, diabetes mellitus, optic atrophy and deafness) syndrome, a rare condition that is usually diagnosed when type 1 diabetes mellitus (DM) presents in childhood. The inheritance is autosomal recessive and the diabetes insipidus tends to develop after the diagnosis of type 1 DM

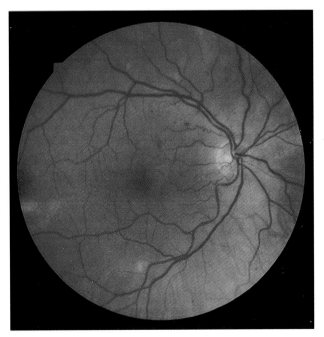

Figure 83 Background diabetic retinopathy with occasional scattered microaneurysms and dot hemorrhages

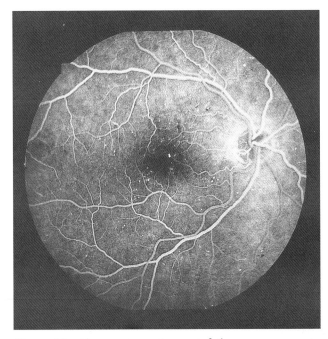

Figure 84 Fluorescein angiogram of the same area as in Figure 83 reveals many more abnormalities than can be seen on the fundal photograph. Widespread microaneurysms appear as white dots

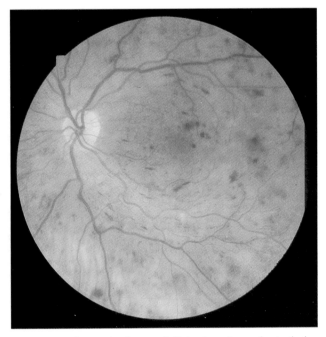

Figure 85 Severe background diabetic retinopathy includes venous changes, clusters and large blot hemorrhages, intraretinal microvascular abnormalities (IRMA), an early cottonwool spot and a generally ischemic appearance. This type of retinopathy is usually a prelude to proliferative change

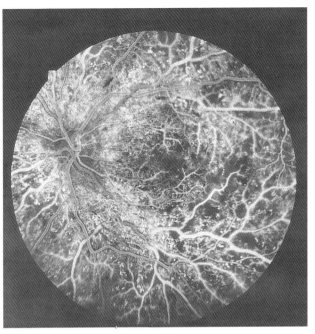

Figure 86 Fluorescein angiogram of the same area as in Figure 85 shows the blind ends of occluded small vessels, widespread capillary leakage and areas of non-perfusion

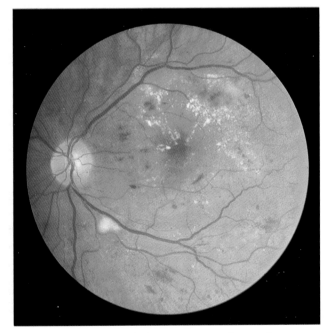

Figure 87 Serious diabetic retinopathy with venous irregularities, blot hemorrhages, intraretinal microvascular abnormalities, large cottonwool spots and extensive areas of hard exudates

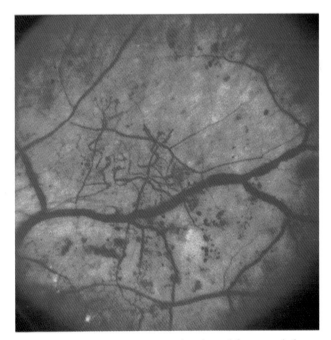

Figure 88 Serious gross peripheral proliferative diabetic retinopathy includes marked venous changes such as dilatation and beading

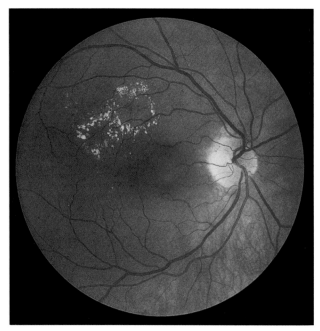

Figure 89 Circinate exudative retinopathy. The two hard exudate rings (lateral to the macula) are true exudates due to leakage from abnormal vessels and are associated with retinal edema. When hard exudates and retinal edema affect the macular area, the fovea may become involved, which may threaten central vision. Laser photocoagulation helps to prevent such loss of vision

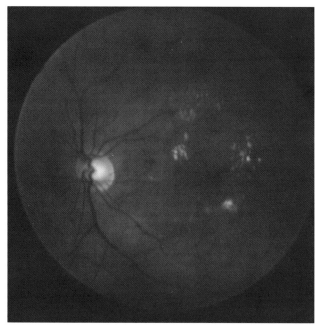

Figure 90 This retinal photograph shows the picture of diabetic maculopathy with frequent hard exudates around the macula immediately prior to intravitreal triamcinolone therapy

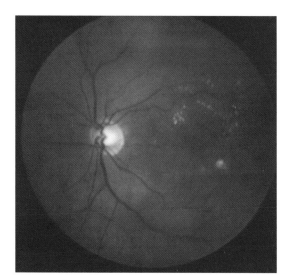

Figure 92 The same retina as in Figure 90 at 3 months post intravitreal triamcinolone therapy. The changes are not dramatic, but there is an improvement with partial resolution of hard exudates around the macula. The role of intravitreal triamcinolone therapy has not been fully established; however, some retina specialists use it to treat diabetic macular edema which persists despite laser therapy. It is not a substitute for laser therapy and one recent study showed it had only a marginal benefit over the long term, while increasing the incidence of cataract and glaucoma

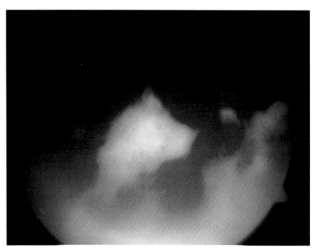

Figure 91 Triamcinolone has been inserted into the vitreous under topical anesthesia

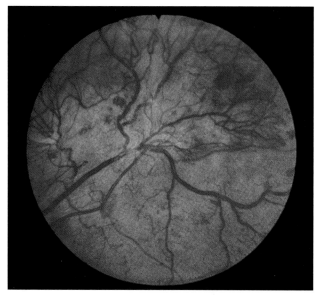

Figure 93 Extensive peripheral proliferative retinopathy with venous beading and blot hemorrhages. New vessels usually originate from a major vein and adopt a branching pattern. Proliferative retinopathy is the most common sight-threatening complication of type 1 diabetes mellitus (DM), with visual loss being due to breakage of vessels leading to preretinal or vitreous hemorrhage. It is always accompanied by other diabetic lesions and is treatable by laser photocoagulation. It is less common in type 2 DM (where exudative maculopathy is the most common cause of visual loss)

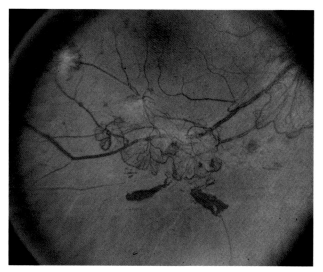

Figure 94 Leashes of peripheral new vessels with associated hemorrhage. These lesions are amenable to laser photocoagulation

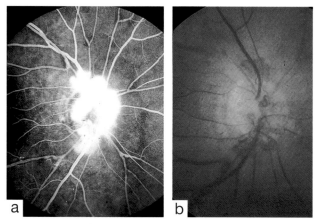

Figure 95 Fluorescein angiogram (a) and fundal photograph (b) of new vessels at the optic disc, which lead rapidly to visual loss. If hemorrhage has already occurred, then visual loss is imminent and urgent laser treatment is indicated. Fluorescein angiography reveals the gross leakage from the abnormal vessels

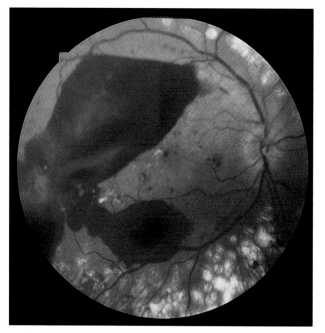

Figure 96 Vitreous hemorrhage has occurred despite extensive laser photocoagulation. The hemorrhage may clear but, if it fails to do so or recurrent hemorrhage ensues, visual loss is inevitable and vitreoretinal surgery may be indicated

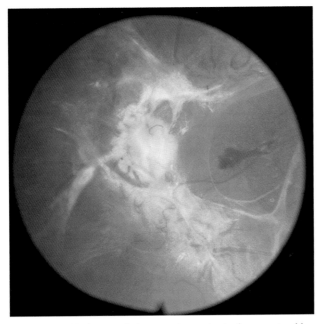

Figure 97 End-stage diabetic retinopathy is characterized by gross distortion of the retina with extensive fibrous bands. Uncontrolled new vessels develop a fibrous tissue covering and expanding fibrous tissue tends to contract, causing retinal traction and detachment. The result is sudden and unexpected visual loss. The retinopathy shown here is untreatable

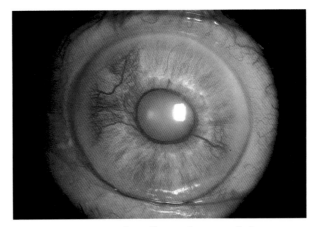

Figure 98 In profoundly ischemic diabetic eyes, thromboneovascular glaucoma may occur with new vessel and fibrous tissue proliferation in the angle of the anterior chamber, which interferes with normal aqueous drainage. The condition is associated with rubeosis iridis (shown here) wherein new vessel growth occurs on the iris

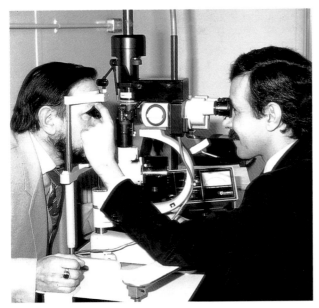

Figure 99 A patient undergoing laser photocoagulation for diabetic retinopathy. A high-energy light beam is focused through a corneal contact lens onto the target area of the retina. Laser photocoagulation can be used to destroy specific targets (e.g. peripheral new vessels) or to perform panretinal photocoagulation

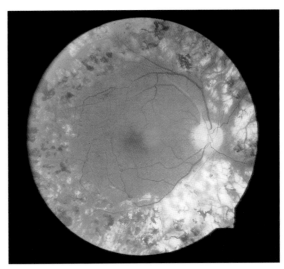

Figure 100 Panretinal laser photocoagulation. The entire retina is treated except for the macula and papillomacular bundle, which are essential for central vision. The rationale for using photocoagulation in proliferative retinopathy is that it destroys the ischemic areas of retina which produce vasoproliferative factors that stimulate new vessel growth. Panretinal photocoagulation may require 1500–2000 burns. The treatment is well tolerated and divided into several sessions, and regression of new vessels is usually seen within 3–4 weeks. Once treatment is effective, the results are long-lasting. In maculopathy, laser treatment is either focused on discrete lesions or uses a diffuse 'grid' treatment in cases of widespread capillary leakage and non-perfusion. However, treatment is less effective and the long-term outlook is not as good

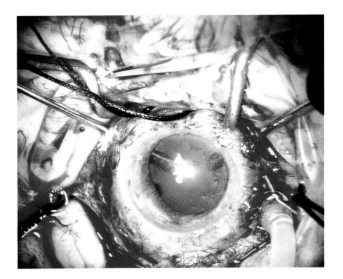

Figure 101 Severe vitreous hemorrhage may lead to secondary retinal detachment. Although vitrectomy may be performed electively for severe vitreous hemorrhage alone, urgent surgery is required for operable retinal detachment. Vitreoretinal microsurgery requires a closed intraocular approach (shown here). An operating microscope allows precise intraocular manipulation to remove the vitreous and its contained hemorrhage, which is replaced with saline and followed by endolaser photocoagulation to prevent both further detachment and subsequent neovascularization

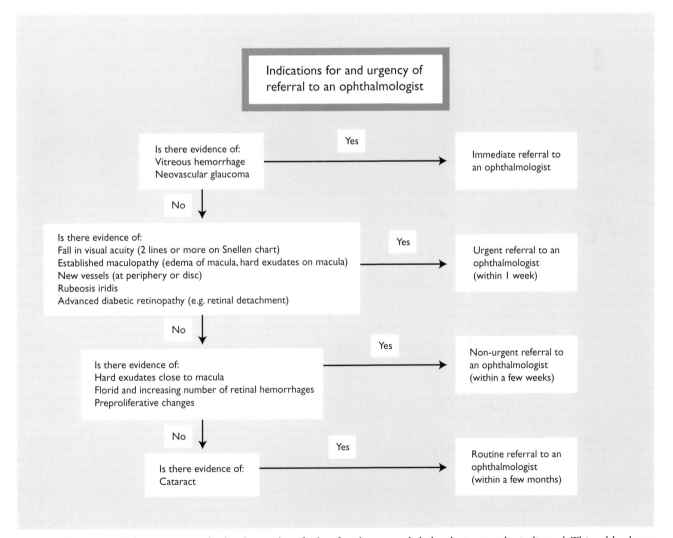

Figure 102 Once diabetic retinopathy has been identified, referral to an ophthalmologist may be indicated. This table shows the types of diabetic eye disease requiring such referral and the urgency with which it should be undertaken

A classification of diabetic neuropathies

Symmetrical polyneuropathies
Symmetrical diffuse sensorimotor neuropathy
Painful small-fiber neuropathy
Acute painful diabetic polyneuropathy

Autonomic neuropathy

Focal and multifocal neuropathy
Entrapment and compression neuropathies
Cranial nerve palsies

Proximal motor neuropathy
(Diabetic amyotrophy)

Hyperglycemic neuropathy

Figure 103 Diabetic neuropathy is a common and often disabling complication of diabetes. Distal symmetric polyneuropathy is the most common form of diabetic neuropathy and can be either sensory or motor and involve small fibers, large fibers or both. Large-fiber neuropathies can involve sensory or motor nerves or both resulting in abnormalities of motor function, vibration perception, position sense and cold thermal perception with commonly a 'glove and stocking' distribution of sensory loss. Small-fiber neuropathy is manifest by pain and paraesthesiae but may develop into a chronic painful neuropathy. Mononeuropathies and entrapment syndromes are common. Proximal motor neuropathies (diabetic amyotrophy) have more complex etiologies but are usually associated with great pain and disability. Autonomic neuropathy is rare and leads to a wide variety of symptoms correlating with the affected autonomic nerve damage. After 20 years of diabetes, around 40% of patients will have diabetic neuropathy

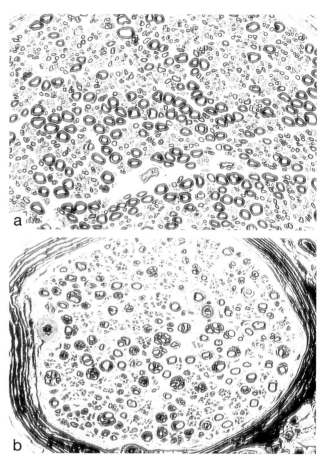

Figure 104 Transverse semi-thin sections of resin-embedded sural nerve biopsy specimens stained with thionin and acridine orange. (a) appearance of a normal nerve. (b) nerve from a patient with diabetic neuropathy shows loss of myelinated nerve fibers and the presence of regenerative clusters. The walls of the endoneural capillaries are thickened. Diabetic neuropathy is a common complication that usually manifests as a sensory, motor or combined symmetrical polyneuropathy. Acute painful neuropathy and diabetic amyotrophy both cause acute pain in the thighs or legs associated with muscle wasting and weight loss. Painful neuropathy may respond to tricyclic drugs, especially amitriptyline, or anticonvulsants, such as gabapentin

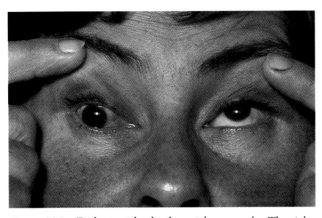

Figure 105 Diabetic right third cranial nerve palsy. The right eye is deviated outwards and downwards, and there is associated ptosis. Pupillary sparing is often encountered. Third nerve palsy is the most commonly seen cranial neuropathy of diabetes, although fourth, sixth and seventh nerve lesions have also been reported as well as intercostal and phrenic nerve lesions. These lesions usually improve over time

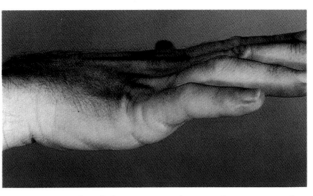

Figure 106 This diabetic patient has an ulnar neuropathy. Such entrapment neuropathies are commonly seen in diabetic patients, the commonest being carpal tunnel syndrome. It has been postulated that diabetic nerves may be more susceptible to mechanical injury

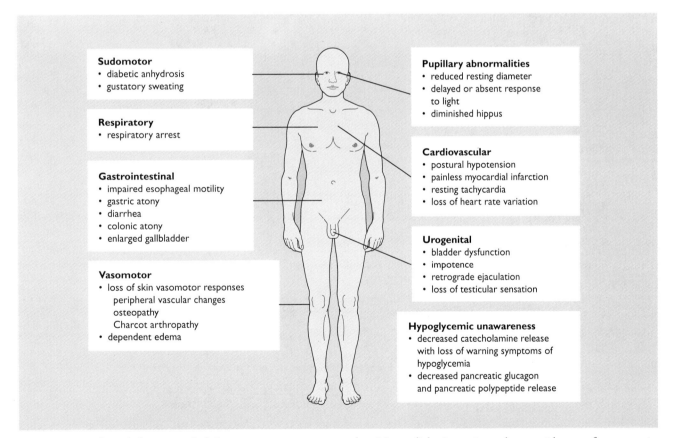

Sudomotor
• diabetic anhydrosis
• gustatory sweating

Respiratory
• respiratory arrest

Gastrointestinal
• impaired esophageal motility
• gastric atony
• diarrhea
• colonic atony
• enlarged gallbladder

Vasomotor
• loss of skin vasomotor responses
    peripheral vascular changes
    osteopathy
    Charcot arthropathy
• dependent edema

Pupillary abnormalities
• reduced resting diameter
• delayed or absent response to light
• diminished hippus

Cardiovascular
• postural hypotension
• painless myocardial infarction
• resting tachycardia
• loss of heart rate variation

Urogenital
• bladder dysfunction
• impotence
• retrograde ejaculation
• loss of testicular sensation

Hypoglycemic unawareness
• decreased catecholamine release with loss of warning symptoms of hypoglycemia
• decreased pancreatic glucagon and pancreatic polypeptide release

Figure 107 Clinical features of diabetic autonomic neuropathy. Many diabetic patients have evidence of autonomic dysfunction, but very few have autonomic symptoms. The most prominent symptom is postural hypotension. Erectile dysfunction, common in diabetic men, is not always due to autonomic neuropathy. Late manifestations other than postural hypotension include gustatory sweating, diabetic diarrhea, gastric atony and reduced awareness of hypoglycemia. Symptomatic autonomic neuropathy may be associated with a poor prognosis

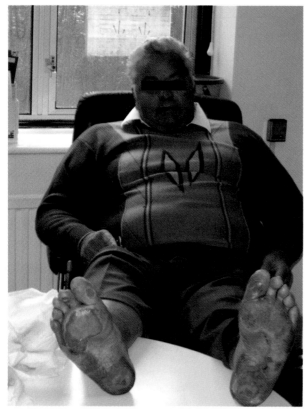

Figure 108 This diabetic patient had known diabetic neuropathy and had been repeatedly given foot care advice in his diabetes center. Despite this, he walked over a hot surface in a Mediterranean country in a summer month. By the time he realized that there was a problem he had sustained extensive burn injuries to both feet requiring urgent medical attention

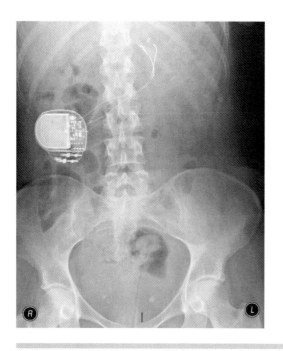

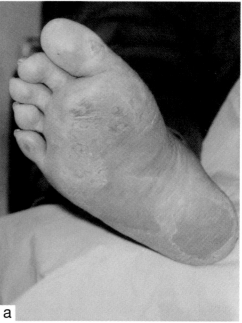

a

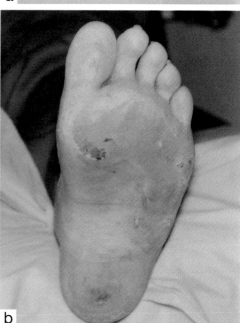

b

Figure 109 In spite of his diabetes and neuropathy and with good care from the podiatrist, this patient's burns healed remarkably quickly, fortunately with no adverse sequelae

Figure 110 Intractable vomiting due to diabetic gastroparesis is notoriously difficult to treat. This patient was successfully treated by the surgical implantation of the Enterra™ Gastric Neurostimulator (GES) system (Medtronic Inc, Minneapolis, USA). This novel experimental approach may prove to be an effective treatment strategy in such rare but difficult-to-treat patients

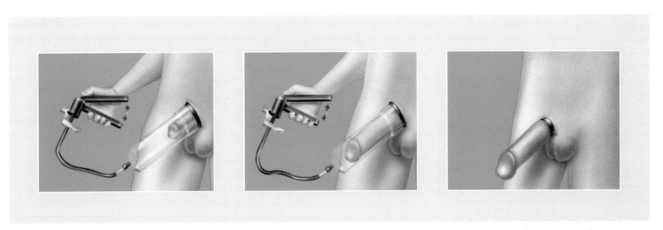

Figure 111 A vacuum system for management of diabetic impotence. Placing the cylinder over the penis and creating a vacuum with the pump produces an erection which can be maintained by placing constrictor rings over the base of the penis. Studies have shown that many patients prefer this non-invasive technique to other, more invasive, methods

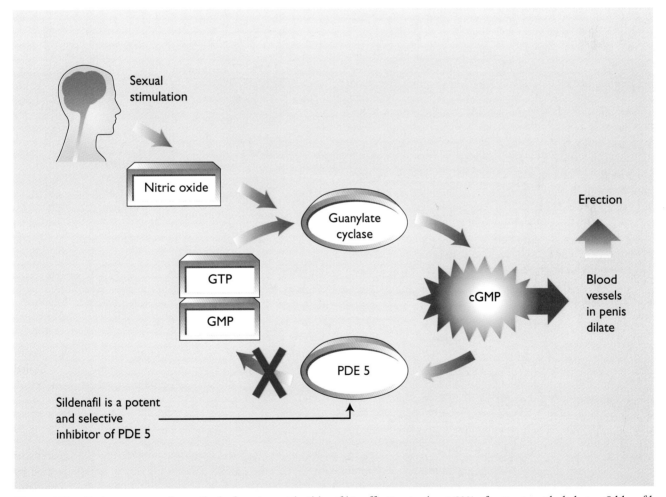

Figure 112 Oral treatment of erectile dysfunction with sildenafil is effective in about 60% of patients with diabetes. Sildenafil selectively inhibits phosphodiesterase type 5 (PDE 5), thereby increasing levels of cyclic GMP within the corpora cavernosa. This enhances the natural erectile response to sexual stimulation

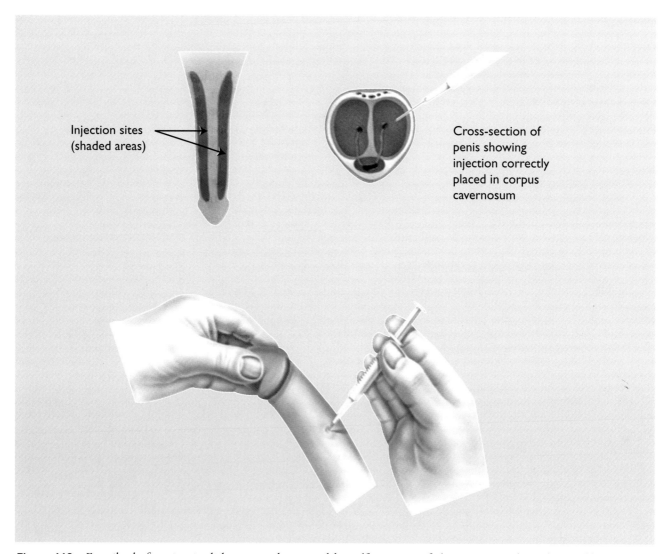

Injection sites (shaded areas)

Cross-section of penis showing injection correctly placed in corpus cavernosum

Figure 113 Erectile dysfunction in diabetes may be treated by self-injection of the vasoactive drug alprostadil (Caverject, Pharmacia, Peapack, NJ, USA) prostaglandin E_1 into the corpus cavernosum of the penis. The resultant smooth muscle relaxation allows increased blood flow into the penis, and penile erection will occur whether or not sexual stimulation is present

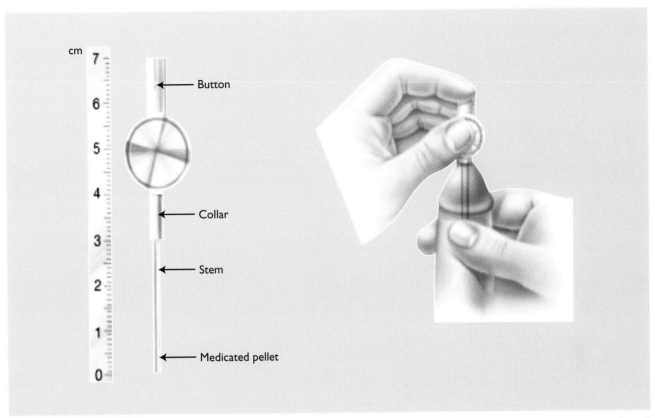

Figure 114 An alternative method of administering alprostadil is by transurethral application of a narrow (1.4 mm) pellet of synthetic prostaglandin E$_1$ directly into the male urethra. Although this removes the need to inject alprostadil, there is still an incidence of penile pain, and controversy exists as to the efficacy of this procedure

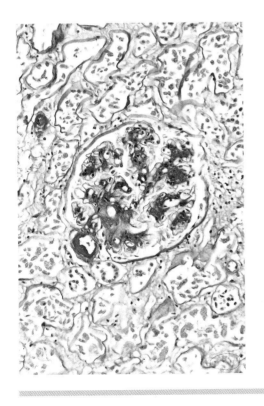

Figure 115 Hyalin deposition in the glomerular tuft in a patient with diabetic glomerulopathy. Other characteristic histopathologic changes of diabetic nephropathy are an increase in glomerular volume, basement membrane thickening and diffuse mesangial enlargement (often with nodular periodic acid-Schiff-positive lesions). Diabetic nephropathy develops in around 35% of type 1 diabetes mellitus (DM) cases and in less than 20% of type 2 DM cases. It is defined as persistent proteinuria (albumin excretion rate > 300 mg/day) associated with hypertension and a falling glomerular filtration rate. Established nephropathy is preceded by years of microalbuminuria (albumin excretion rate 30–300 mg/day) which is negative on reagent-strip testing for albumin. Vigorous control of blood pressure and the use of angiotensin-converting enzyme inhibitors have been shown to delay the rate of progression of diabetic nephropathy. Periodic acid-Schiff stain

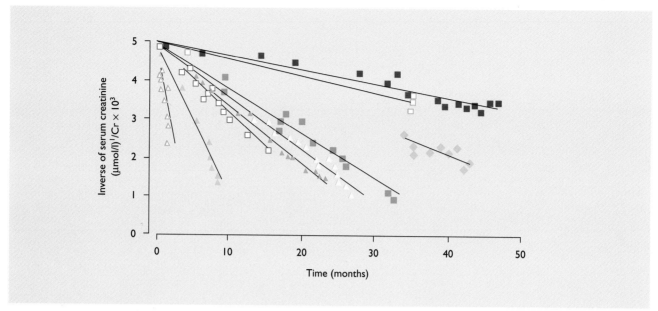

Figure 116 Once renal failure has become established in diabetes, there is an inexorable decline in renal function which, if untreated, leads to end-stage renal failure. The decline in renal function is linear when plotted as the inverse of serum creatinine over time. Modern treatment strategies attempt to slow the deterioration of renal function by vigorous anti-hypertensive regimens. Angiotensin-converting enzyme inhibitors may be especially effective because they reduce intraglomerular pressure and, unless renal failure is advanced, it is still worthwhile to attempt to achieve improved glycemic control

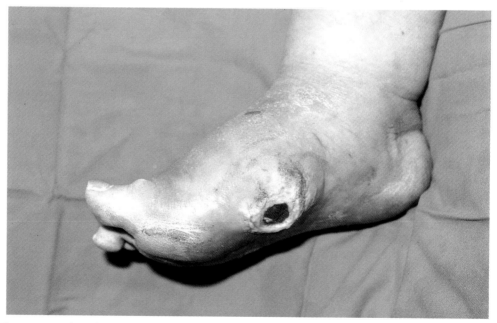

Figure 117 This neuropathic ulcer on the medial aspect of the foot in a diabetic patient shows the characteristic punched-out appearance on heavily calloused skin. The neuropathic foot is numb, warm and dry with palpable pulses. Charcot arthropathy complicates the neuropathic foot and presents with warmth, swelling and redness (shown here). Ulceration occurs at areas of high pressure in the deformed foot, especially over the metatarsal heads. Minor trauma such as ill-fitting or new shoes, or the presence of a small undetected object in the shoe, can result in serious foot ulceration. Treatment is by bedrest, debridement and appropriate antibiotics to treat secondary infection. Special shoes and plaster casts (to allow mobility while taking pressure off the ulcer) are also useful

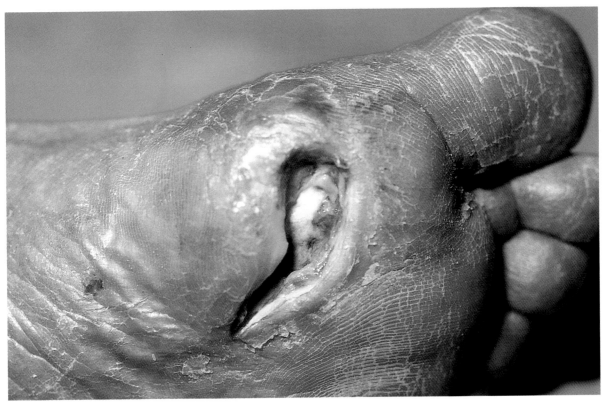

Figure 118 Deeply penetrating diabetic neuropathic ulcer over the metatarsal head caused by a foreign body. Foot education, especially in those patients with documented neuropathy, is essential for preventing such lesions and should be undertaken by chiropodists, diabetic specialist nurses and diabetic physicians. Diabetic patients should not put their feet in front of fires or on radiators. Their feet should also be regularly inspected for early ulceration and their shoes carefully checked for foreign objects before being worn

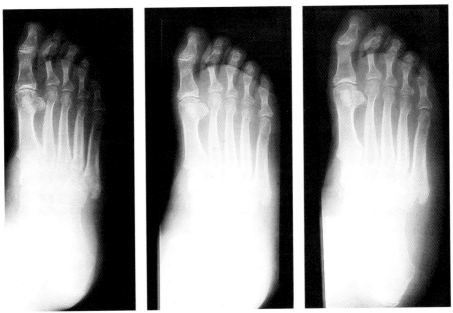

Figure 119 Three radiographs of the same neuropathic foot taken 1 month apart. Progressive damage to the foot has led to complete disorganization of the midtarsal joints without osteoporosis. These are typical appearances of a Charcot joint

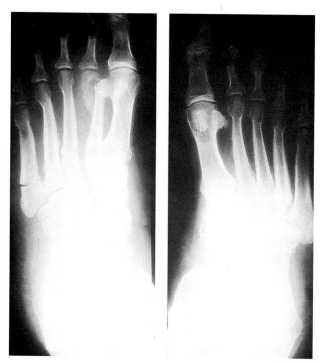

Figure 120 Radiographs of the feet of a diabetic patient showing a neuropathic ulcer over the metatarsal heads of the left foot. Destruction of the left second metatarsal head and associated soft-tissue swelling are secondary to osteomyelitis complicating the ulcer. A fracture on the base of the fifth metatarsal is also present. The right foot shows Charcot disorganization of the midtarsal joints

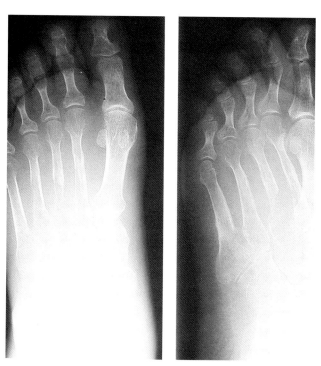

Figure 121 Osteomyelitis in the diabetic foot with destruction of the base of the third metatarsal (right) and a periosteal reaction in the shafts of the adjacent metatarsals accompanied by osteoporosis

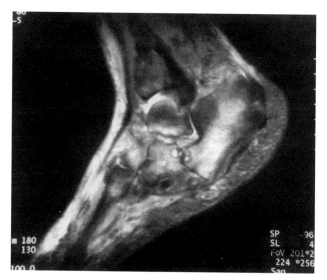

Figure 122 Sagittal magnetic resonance image of the hind foot of a diabetic patient showing marrow edema of the calcaneus consistent with acute osteomyelitis. There is also fluid deep to the plantar fascia consistent with cellulitis. An ankle effusion is also present

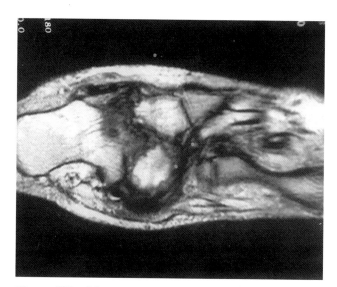

Figure 123 Magnetic resonance image of a diabetic foot showing disorganization of the talo-calcaneonavicular joint with erosions of the articular surface. Such appearances in a diabetic patient are typical of a Charcot joint

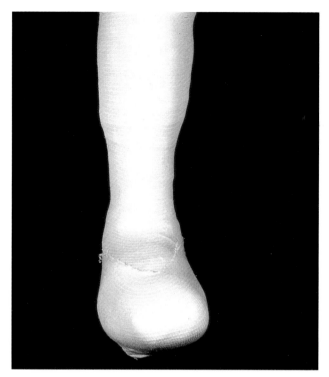

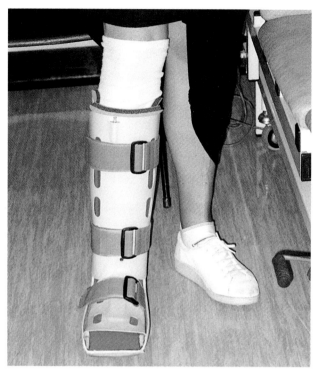

Figure 124 The reduction of weight-bearing forces is an essential part of the treatment of significant neuropathic ulceration and can be achieved, on a short-term basis, by the use of a total-contact lightweight plaster cast designed to unload pressure from the ulcer and other vulnerable areas while allowing continued mobility. For the long term, however, equal redistribution of weight-bearing forces over the sole of the foot is achieved by the use of special footwear and insoles

Figure 125 Off-loading pressure from diabetic foot ulcers is essential to allow healing. Total contact plaster casts may be used, but are not free from problems. A more recent alternative is the Aircast Pneumatic Walker™ with a Diabetic Conversion Kit. It is a light-weight removable plastic brace lined with inflatable chambers to promote off-loading. Experience to date has shown that such a boot greatly increases the immediate off-loading capacity of the diabetic foot clinic

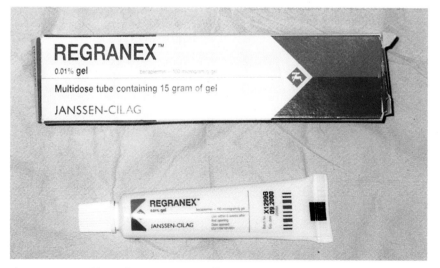

Figure 126 A topical preparation of becaplermin (Regranex™) has been recently introduced as an adjunct in the treatment of full-thickness, neuropathic, diabetic foot ulcers. Becaplermin is recombinant human platelet-derived growth factor. Experience to date with this product is limited and it is very expensive. Accurate cost–benefit analyses are awaited

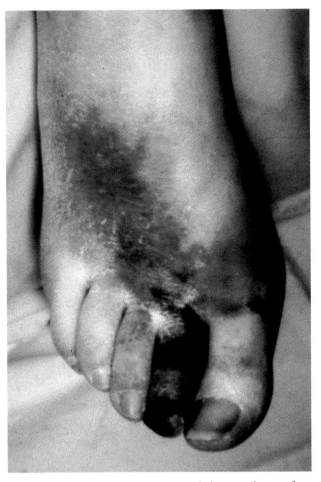

Figure 127 Distal gangrene in a diabetic ischemic foot (dorsal view)

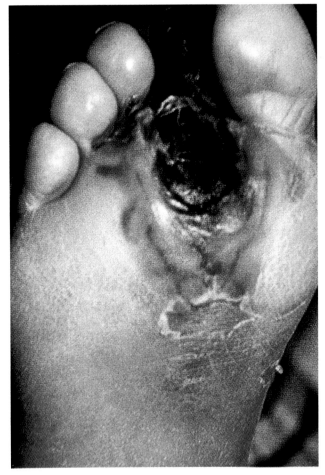

Figure 128 Plantar view of the same foot as in Figure 127 shows the common diabetic complications of ischemia and neuropathy, both of which may lead to ulceration. The ischemic foot is cold, pulseless and subject to rest pain, ulceration and gangrene (shown here). Ischemic ulceration usually affects the margins of the foot and may be amenable to angioplasty or reconstructive arterial surgery

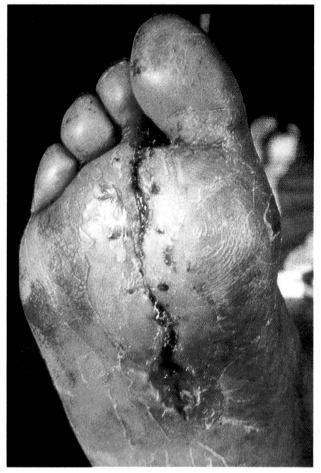

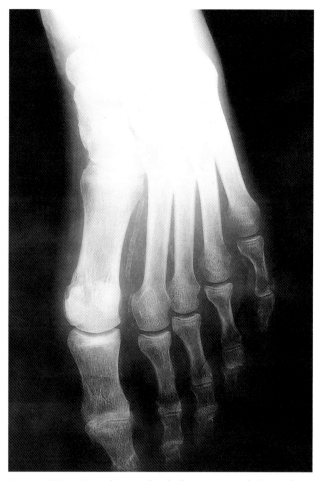

Figure 129 The same foot as in Figures 127 and 128 after amputation of the second toe. A good result has been obtained. However, a large proportion of diabetic patients with critical ischemia or gangrene of the lower limbs undergo major amputation. Thus, the importance of adequate screening and preventive measures to avoid these operations cannot be overemphasized

Figure 130 Digital arterial calcification in a diabetic foot. Peripheral vascular disease is a particularly common vascular complication of diabetes and about half of all lower limb amputations involve diabetic patients

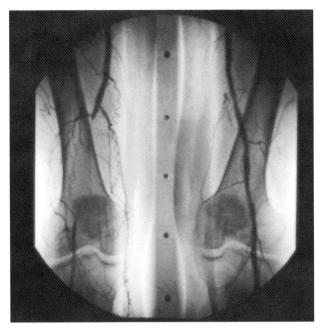

Figure 131 Angiogram showing occlusion of the right popliteal artery at the adductor canal in a diabetic patient with peripheral vascular disease (left). There are many collateral vessels and the artery reconstitutes distally below the knee. The opposite side (right), which is normal, is shown for comparison

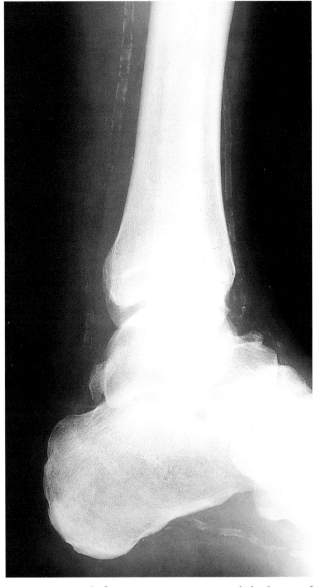

Figure 132 Calcification accompanying medial sclerosis of the distal lower limb arteries. In diabetes, the distal blood vessels are often affected by both atheroma and medial sclerosis with calcification. This must be borne in mind if reconstructive vascular surgery or percutaneous transluminal balloon angioplasty is contemplated for symptomatic peripheral vascular disease. The initial success rate with angioplasty is reduced in diabetic patients

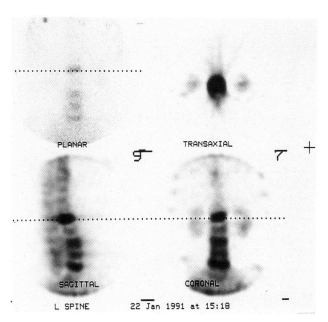

Figure 134 Bone scan showing osteoporotic vertebral collapse in a patient with type 1 diabetes mellitus, which has been associated with a generalized reduction in bone density (diabetic osteopenia). It is probably more common in those patients exhibiting poor metabolic control and is due to reduced bone formation rather than increased resorption. A slightly increased risk of susceptibility to fracture results from this abnormality

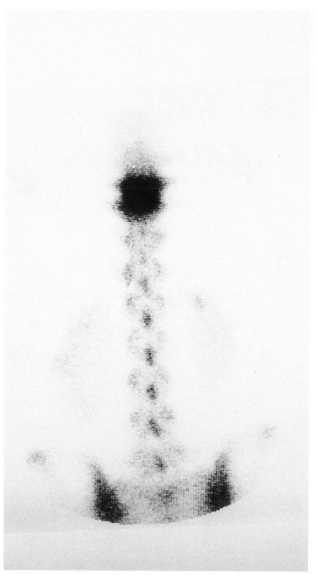

Figure 133 Bone scan of the spine (posterior view) in a poorly controlled type 2 diabetes mellitus patient shows the florid increase in activity in adjacent vertebrae typical of osteomyelitis

The skin in diabetes

Necrobiosis lipoidica diabeticorum
Diabetic dermopathy
Diabetic bullae
Bacterial and *Candida* infection
Acanthosis nigricans
Vitiligo
Eruptive xanthomata
Necrolytic migratory erythema
Insulin allergy
Lipoatrophy
Lipohypertrophy

Figure 135 Many abnormalities of the skin are found in diabetic patients. Some may not be specific to diabetes. Acanthosis nigricans is a skin manifestation of insulin resistant states, while vitiligo is a cutaneous marker of autoimmunity. Eruptive xanthomata are associated with significant hypertriglyceridemia. Necrolytic migratory erythema occurs in patients with a glucagonoma and associated diabetes and is very rare. The rashes of insulin allergy, lipoatrophy and lipohypertrophy are all associated with exogenous insulin administration

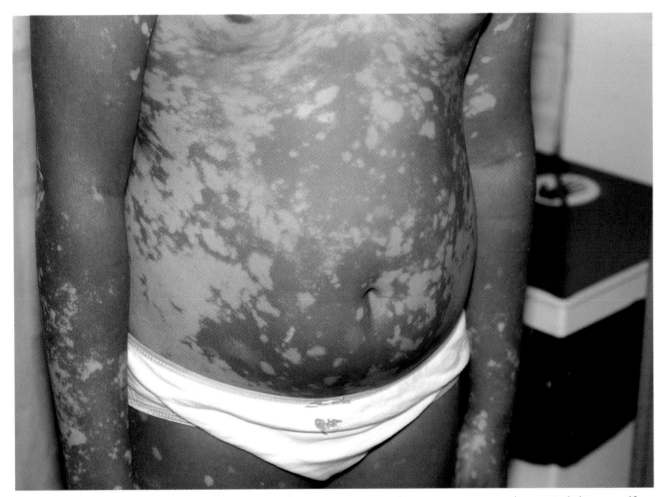

Figure 136 Vitiligo, autoimmune destruction of melanocytes, is commonly seen in patients with type 1 diabetes, itself an autoimmune condition

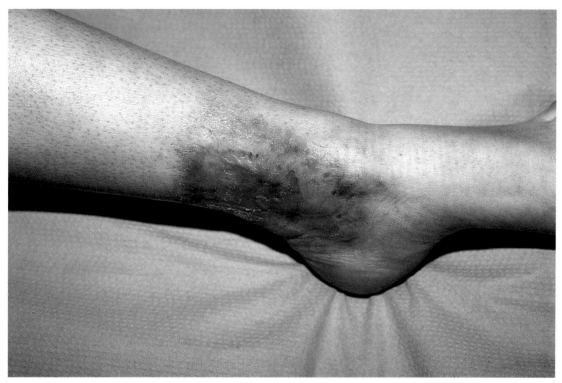

Figure 137 A typical lesion of necrobiosis lipoidica diabeticorum on the shin. These lesions are usually non-scaling plaques with yellow atrophic centers and an erythematous edge, and predominantly affect diabetic women. They vary considerably in size, and are often multiple and bilateral. Necrobiosis may occur in non-diabetic subjects

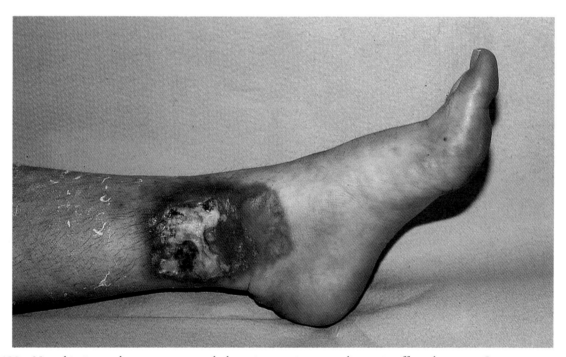

Figure 138 Necrobiosis may become severe and ulcerative, causing great distress in affected patients. Spontaneous regression may occur and treatment tends to be unsatisfactory. Skin grafts may become complicated by recurrence within the graft or at an adjacent site

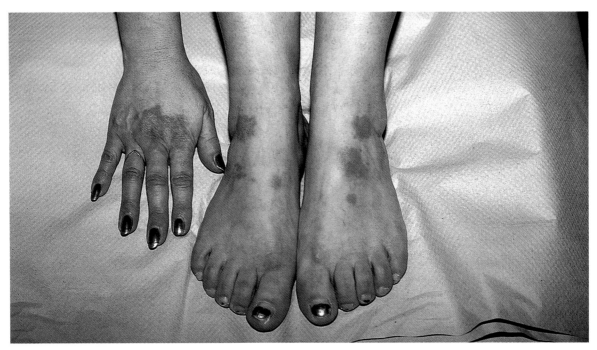

Figure 139 Granuloma annulare. Although this skin condition is occasionally seen in diabetic patients, several large studies have failed to reveal a significant association between the two disorders, both of which are relatively common

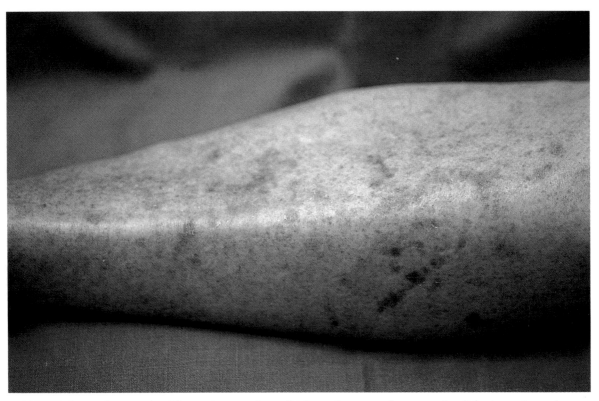

Figure 140 Diabetic dermopathy. These pigmented pretibial patches are often seen in diabetic patients, but are not pathognomonic of the disease. There is a male preponderance and the lesions are discrete, atrophic, scaly or hyperpigmented. The underlying cause is not known

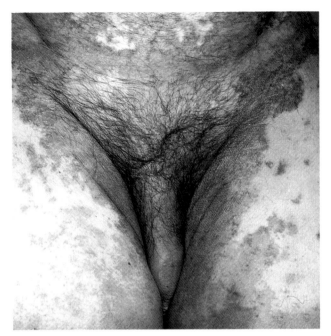

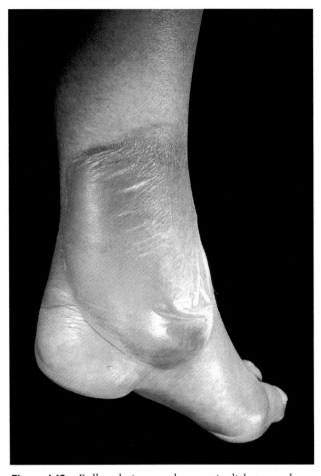

Figure 141 Migratory necrolytic erythema. This rash is associated with glucagon-secreting pancreatic tumors (or occasionally zinc deficiency). Such rashes tend to wax and wane in cycles of 1–2 weeks. Diabetes is presumed to be due to increased glucagon-stimulated hepatic gluconeogenesis. Weight loss, diarrhea and mood changes are frequent features, but death is usually due to massive venous thrombosis. Treatment is by zinc supplementation, or somatostatin or a somatostatin analog

Figure 142 Bullous lesions rarely occur in diabetes, and can only be diagnosed when other bullous disorders have been excluded. They usually occur suddenly with no obvious history of trauma and may take a long time to heal. The lower legs and feet are usually affected, and there is a male preponderance

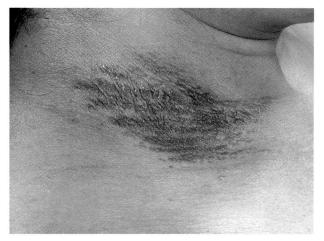

Figure 143 Acanthosis nigricans is uncommon. These brown hyperkeratotic plaques with a velvety surface occur most frequently in the axillae and flexures, and on the neck. Acanthosis is associated with insulin resistance caused by genetic defects in the insulin receptor or postreceptor function, or the presence of antibodies to the insulin receptor

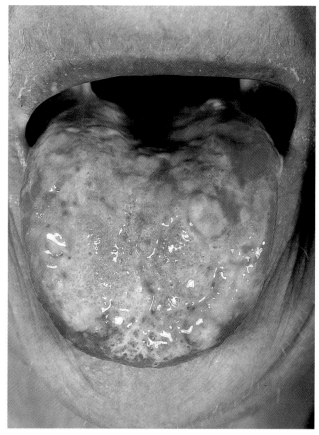

Figure 144 Candidiasis is a common fungal infection in diabetic patients. Although particularly common in the vagina or perineum (pruritus vulvae), under the breasts (intertrigo) and on the tip of the penis (balanitis), it may occur elsewhere. The yeasts thrive in glucose-containing media and, hence, control of blood-glucose levels helps to eradicate this troublesome infection. Antifungal creams may be necessary until glucose levels are controlled, but oral antifungal agents are rarely required

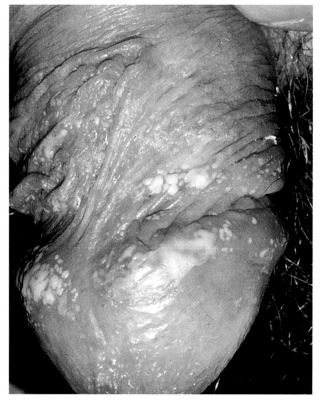

Figure 145 Balanitis secondary to diabetes mellitus is a candidal infection of the distal end of the penis and is common at the time of presentation of diabetes in men

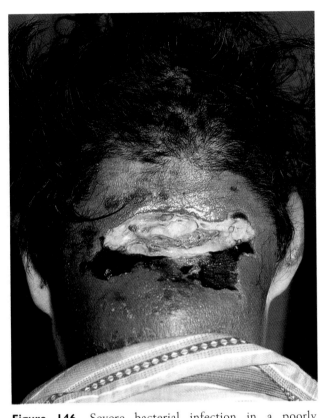

Figure 146 Severe bacterial infection in a poorly controlled diabetic patient. Although it is widely believed that diabetic patients are more prone to infection than non-diabetic subjects, it is unclear whether diabetic patients have an increase in the rate of infection in general. Diabetic patients are susceptible to certain infections, including tuberculosis, urinary tract infections and infections due to unusual micro-organisms such as osteomyelitis, mucor-mycosis and enterococcal meningitis. Diabetes is thought to impair several aspects of cellular function necessary to combat infection

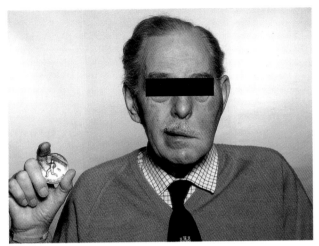

Figure 147 Malignant otitis externa. This infection, which can be extremely serious, is almost always due to *Pseudomonas* species, as was the case here. Affected patients usually have poorly controlled diabetes. This elderly diabetic patient has a seventh cranial nerve palsy as a complication. Antipseudomonal antibiotics and an early surgical opinion are advised

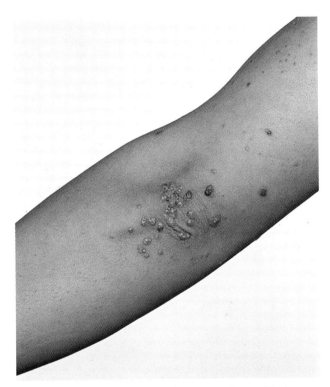

Figure 148 Eruptive xanthomata. Type V hyper-lipoproteinemia with an increase in very-low-density lipoproteins (VLDLs) and chylomicrons is often associated with glucose intolerance. This lipoprotein abnormality is accentuated by obesity and alcohol consumption, and may lead to acute pancreatitis and peripheral neuropathy

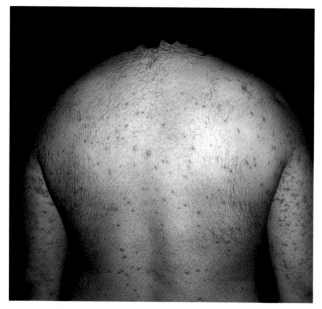

Figure 149 Massive eruptive xanthomata in a young man with type 2 diabetes mellitus

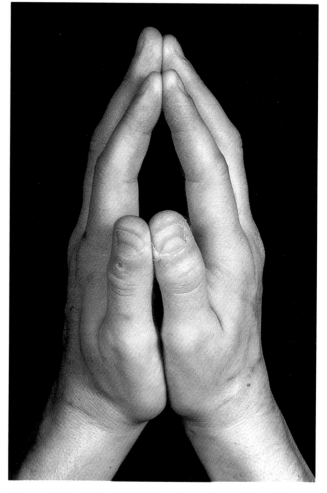

Figure 150 Diabetic cheiroarthropathy or limited joint mobility is characterized by an inability to extend fully the metacarpophalangeal and proximal interphalangeal joints when the tips of the fingers and palms of the hands are opposed in the so-called prayer sign. Although it may be seen in adult-onset type 1 and 2 diabetes mellitus (DM), it is most commonly seen in children and young adults with type 1 DM. The development of this abnormality is linked to the duration of diabetes. When present, other diabetic complications are likely to coexist

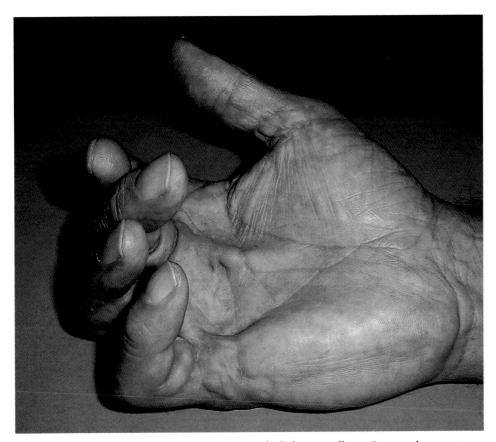

Figure 151 Dupuytren's contracture is common in patients with diabetes mellitus. Conversely, in patients presenting with Dupuytren's contracture, a high prevalence of diabetes is found. The exact nature of the link between the two conditions remains unclear

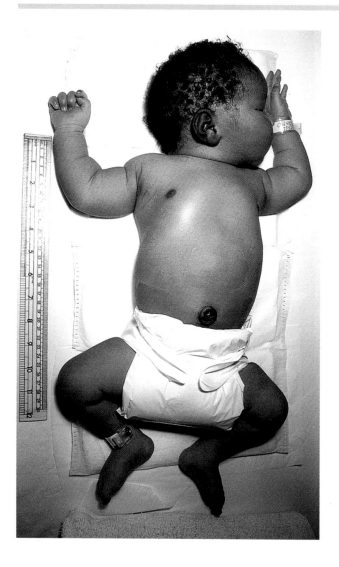

Figure 152 Macrosomic baby of a diabetic mother. In diabetic women, blood concentrations of fuel substrates (glucose, amino acids and fatty acids) are raised and their delivery to the fetus increased. The elevated glucose and amino-acid levels stimulate fetal β-cells to hypersecrete insulin. The increased insulin secretion and nutrient availability promote fetal growth which, in turn, leads to macrosomia. Vaginal delivery may be impossible in cases of gross macrosomia. Strict glycemic control is mandatory in diabetic pregnancy and requires frequent attendance at a joint obstetric/antenatal clinic. The increased motivation of pregnancy appears to help most diabetic mothers achieve excellent diabetic control

8 Diabetic dyslipidemia

Lipid disorders assume a position of utmost importance in patients with diabetes because of the high risk of macrovascular disease in this condition. Patients with well controlled type 1 diabetes mellitus (DM) have lipoprotein concentrations similar to the background non-diabetic population. With poor control, increased concentrations of triglyceride-rich lipoproteins are seen giving rise to hypertriglyceridemia. The most common lipoprotein abnormality in type 2 diabetes is an elevation in triglycerides and very-low-density lipoprotein (VLDL) caused by an overproduction of VLDL triglyceride. Lipoprotein lipase activity is probably decreased in type 2 diabetes, possibly as a manifestation of insulin resistance, and this may be a direct cause of elevated VLDL levels. No consistent changes in low-density lipoprotein (LDL) cholesterol are seen in type 2 diabetes, but a number of potentially atherogenic changes in LDL composition have been observed particularly a predominance of small dense LDL particles. The finding of decreased high-density lipoprotein (HDL) concentrations is very prevalent in type 2 diabetes adding to the atherogenic lipid profile of this disorder. No consistent change in lipoprotein a (Lp(a)) concentrations has been found in type 2 diabetes.

Evidence is accumulating that patients with type 2 DM benefit at least as much as non-diabetic subjects from statin therapy. Simvastatin treated patients with diabetes in the Scandinavian Simvastatin Survival Study (4S Trial) exhibited reductions in major coronary events and revascularization procedures of 42% and 48%, respectively. In the Cholesterol and Recurrent Events Trial (CARE), pravastatin therapy reduced the incidence of recurrent coronary heart disease (CHD) events (CHD death, non-fatal myocardial infarction, coronary artery bypass graft and revascularization) by 25%. There were 586 patients with diabetes in this study. In the Veterans Affairs HDL Intervention Trial (VA-HIT), gemfibrozil was used as secondary prevention. Patients had documented CHD with low HDL cholesterol levels and the aim was to study the effect of gemfibrozil on the risk of recurrent CHD events. About half of the patients had either type 2 DM or abdominal obesity and hyperinsulinemia (insulin resistance/metabolic syndrome). Gemfibrozil reduced the risk of myocardial infarction and CHD-related mortality by 22% without any lowering of LDL cholesterol.

The Collaborative Atorvastatin Diabetes Study (CARDS) included 2838 patients with type 2 diabetes and no documented previous history of cardiovascular disease (CVD) with at least one of the following features: retinopathy, albuminuria, current smoking or hypertension. Patients had an LDL cholesterol concentration of 4.14 mmol/l (160 mg/dl) or lower. As compared to a placebo, addition of atorvastatin 10 mg daily led to a 37% reduction in major cardiovascular events and reduced the risk of stroke by 48% with overall a highly statistically significant reduction in the composite primary end point of acute coronary events, coronary revascularization and stroke. A 27% fall in all-cause mortality was also observed, however, this just failed to reach statistical significance.

Patients with type 2 DM are thought to be at the same risk of a CVD event as non-diabetic patients with existing CVD. Lipid-lowering therapy is likely to be as clinically effective and cost-effective in patients with type 2 diabetes who have not yet sustained a cardiovascular event as in non-diabetic subjects with documented CVD.

All adult patients with diabetes should have a fasting lipid profile to assess their lipid status and to search for any lipid disorder that necessitates lipid-lowering treatment. How often this should be done is debatable. The American Diabetes Association (ADA) suggests screening for hyperlipidemia on an annual basis. Lifestyle modification focusing on the reduction of saturated fat and cholesterol intake, weight loss (where indicated) and increased physical activity is recommended for diabetic patients with hyperlipidemia and has been shown to improve the lipid profile. The ADA position statement on lipid disorders is as follows.

Individuals with diabetes who are over the age of 40 years with a total cholesterol $\geq 135 \, mg/dl$ (3.5 mmol/l) without overt CVD should be treated with a statin to achieve an LDL cholesterol reduction of 30–40% regardless of baseline LDL level, and with a primary goal of reducing LDL cholesterol to $< 100 \, mg/dl$ (2.6 mmol/l). Those individuals less than 40 years of age without overt CVD but with cardiovascular risk factors or long duration of diabetes should have lipid-lowering therapy to reduce LDL cholesterol to $< 100 \, mg/dl$ (2.6 mmol/l) if this target is not reached by lifestyle modification alone. Patients with diabetes and overt CVD should all be treated with a statin with an option of a lowered LDL cholesterol target of $< 70 \, mg/dl$ (1.8 mmol/l). Triglycerides should be lowered to $< 150 \, mg/dl$ (1.7 mmol/l) and HDL cholesterol should be raised to $> 40 \, mg/dl$ (1.15 mmol/l). In women, an HDL target of $> 50 \, mg/dl$ should be considered.

High LDL levels should be treated with a statin (hydroxymethylglutaryl-coenzyme A reductase inhibitor) examples of which include simvastatin, atorvastatin, pravastatin and rosuvastatin. The typical dyslipidemia of type 2 DM of raised triglycerides and low HDL cholesterol may respond better to a fibrate, such as fenofibrate, bezafibrate or gemfibrozil. Fibrates bind to the peroxisome proliferator-activated receptor (PPARα) ultimately leading to an interaction with several genes critical to the control of lipid metabolism. Ezetimibe is an extremely potent and specific inhibitor of dietary and biliary cholesterol absorption. In one study, compared to placebo, ezetimibe produced a 15% reduction in total cholesterol, a 20% reduction in LDL cholesterol, an 8% reduction in triglycerides and a 3% rise in HDL cholesterol.

Combination therapy such as statin/fibrate and statin/ezetimibe may be necessary to achieve lipid targets, although more careful monitoring is required as such combinations are likely to be associated with known side-effects of some lipid-lowering agents such as myositis.

BIBLIOGRAPHY

American Diabetes Association. Management of dyslipidemia in adults with diabetes. Diabetes Care 1999; 22 (Suppl 1): 556–9

American Diabetes Association. Clinical Practice Recommendations 2005. Diabetes Care 2005; 28 (Suppl 1): s1–s80

Colhoun HM, Betteridge DJ, Durrington PN, et al. Primary prevention of cardiovascular disease with Atorvastatin in Type 2 diabetes in the Collaborative Atorvastatin Diabetes Study (CARDS): multicentre randomised placebo-controlled trial. Lancet 2004; 36: 685–96

Durrington P. Statins and fibrates in the management of diabetic dyslipidemia. Diabet Med 1997; 14: 513–16

Goldberg RB, Mellies MJ, Sacks FM, et al. Cardiovascular events and their reduction with pravastatin in diabetic and glucose-intolerant myocardial infarction survivors with average cholesterol levels. Circulation 1998; 98: 2513–19

Grover SA, Coupal L, Zowall H, et al. How cost-effective is the treatment of dyslipidemia in patients with diabetes but without cardiovascular disease? Diabetes Care 2001; 24: 45–50

Haffner SM, Alexander CM, Cook TJ, et al. Reduced coronary events in simvastatin-treated patients with coronary heart disease and diabetes or impaired fasting glucose levels: sub-group analyses in the Scandinavian Simvastatin Survival Study. Arch Intern Med 1999; 159: 2661–7

Rubins HB, Robins SJ, Collins D, et al. Gemfibrozil for the secondary prevention of coronary heart disease in men with low levels of high-density lipoprotein cholesterol. Veterans Affairs High-Density Lipoprotein Cholesterol Intervention Trial Study Group. N Engl J Med 1999; 341: 410–18

Steiner G. Lipid intervention trials in diabetes. Diabetes Care 2000; 23 (Suppl 2): B49–53

9   Diabetes and pregnancy

Pregnancy in women with diabetes poses a challenge with potential adverse consequences for both mother and fetus. There is also evidence that children born to a diabetic mother are at increased risk of future obesity and diabetes. As maternal diabetes is hazardous for the fetus with an increased risk of major congenital malformations and metabolic and developmental problems, diabetic patients should be closely supervised during pregnancy and preferably attend a combined diabetic/obstetric clinic. Women with type 1 diabetes who are of reproductive age should be asked about future plans for conception and advised to attempt to normalize their HbA_{1c} levels prior to conception to avoid the risk of congenital malformations (most commonly sacral agenesis).

There is now little excess mortality among diabetic mothers. Perinatal mortality among diabetic pregnancies approaches that for non-diabetic pregnancy, but still remains above that for the general population largely because of stillbirth, congenital malformation and the respiratory distress syndrome that affects infants born prematurely. Other neonatal problems include jaundice, hypoglycemia and polycythemia. Fetal macrosomia leads to problems with delivery (dystocia).

Uncontrolled diabetes may cause fetal loss as a result of early spontaneous miscarriage. The congenital malformation rate of 4–10% remains three to five times greater than that in the general population with malformations involving the heart and central nervous system being potentially lethal. Diabetic malformations are likely to be caused by both genetic and environmental factors with glucose being the most likely major teratogen through an unidentified mechanism. The increase in congenital abnormalities is related to the HbA_{1c} level in early pregnancy hence the importance of pre-pregnancy counseling.

Maternal hyperglycemia in diabetic pregnancy is thought to be the major stimulus for the consequent fetal hyperinsulinemia and resultant abnormal fetal growth. The frequency of large-for-gestational-age infants in diabetes is approximately twice as high as in non-diabetic pregnancies. Such infants are at increased risk of emergency cesarean section, birth trauma and birth asphyxia. There is also an unexplained excess of late stillbirths in diabetic pregnancies. The combined diabetic/obstetric clinic should be staffed by a diabetologist with an interest in obstetrics, an obstetrician with an interest in diabetes, a diabetes specialist nurse, a midwife and a dietician. The mother with type 1 diabetes will need to attend at frequent intervals, usually every 1–2 weeks. An early ultrasound scan is recommended to identify gestational age and search for gross congenital abnormalities. Type 1 diabetic patients who are pregnant need to monitor their blood glucose levels intensively. Frequent adjustments of insulin doses based on the results are undertaken usually on the recommendation of the diabetologist. There is a physiologic decrease in insulin sensitivity between the second and third trimesters of pregnancy, so insulin dose requirements usually increase gradually throughout the second trimester. Appetite is also less affected by the nausea of early pregnancy, so food intake rises. Existing retinopathy may worsen during pregnancy or new retinopathy appear, hence detailed retinal screening is mandatory during the pregnancy. Pregnant mothers with diabetic nephropathy are a high-risk group. Pregnancy may worsen renal function, occasionally irreversibly. A successful outcome of pregnancy is likely when serum creatinine is less than 175 μmol/l and diastolic blood pressure is less than 90 mmHg before conception. Fewer than half the pregnancies are successful when creatinine exceeds 250 μmol/l. Diabetic women who have had a renal or combined renal-pancreatic transplant have had successfully completed pregnancies.

A repeat ultrasound scan should be performed at 18–20 weeks' gestation and regularly after 26 weeks to assess fetal growth and liquor volume. Most specialist centers advocate delivery at 38 weeks, although some may allow women with uncomplicated diabetes to go into spontaneous labor. Respiratory distress syndrome is a major cause of neonatal morbidity and mortality in diabetic pregnancies. It is difficult to predict its occurrence. Pre-eclampsia is also more common in diabetic pregnancy. The mother's diabetes is best managed by continuous intravenous insulin infusion during labor or cesarean section. Following delivery, insulin requirements fall promptly to normal pre-pregnancy levels. The neonates of the diabetic mother may exhibit several abnormalities. These include macrosomia, congenital malformations, hypoglycemia owing to fetal hyperinsulinemia, polycythemia, respiratory distress syndrome, transient hypertrophic cardiomyopathy, hypocalcemia, hypomagnesemia and jaundice. All require skilled assessment and management by the neonatal team.

An increasing number of pregnant patients with type 2 diabetes are being encountered. Many are undiagnosed during the critical stages of organogenesis and have the same high risk of congenital abnormalities as patients with poorly controlled type 1 diabetes. Pregnancies of women with type 2 diabetes may be at even more risk than those with type 1 diabetes owing to poor glycemic control in early pregnancy, obesity, greater age and increased parity.

Gestational diabetes mellitus (GDM) is glucose intolerance first recognized during pregnancy. Occasionally type 1 or type 2 diabetes presents in pregnancy. There is a lack of agreed diagnostic criteria for GDM, but this should not detract from the detrimental impact of maternal hyperglycemia on the pregnancy and the future health of the mother and child. The American Diabetes Association recommends immediate glucose testing for those women deemed to be at

high risk of GDM (marked obesity, previous history of GDM, glycosuria or strong family history of diabetes). A fasting plasma glucose ≥126 mg/dl (7 mmol/l) or a random plasma glucose ≥200 mg/dl (11 mmol/l) meets the threshold for diagnosis of GDM and should be confirmed on a subsequent day. High-risk women not found to have GDM at initial screening and average-risk women should be screened between 24 and 26 weeks of gestation by either a one-step approach using a 100 g oral glucose tolerance test (OGTT) or a two-step approach. The two-step approach involves measuring the plasma glucose 1 h after a 50 g oral glucose load and performing a 100 g OGTT test on those women who exceed the glucose threshold 1h after the 50 g oral glucose load. A glucose threshold value of ≥140 mg/dl (7.8 mg/dl) identifies around 80% of women with GDM. Diagnostic criteria for the 100 g OGTT are as follows: ≥95 mg/dl (5.3 mmol/l) fasting, ≥180 mg/dl (10 mmol/l) at 1 h, ≥155 mg/dl (8.6 mmol/l) at 2 h and ≥140 mg/dl (7.8 mmol/l) at 3 h. Two or more of the plasma glucose values must be met or exceeded to make the diagnosis of GDM. In many other countries, such testing methods are not used and there is a reliance on the 75 g OGTT as recommended by the WHO. GDM is associated with high parity, obesity, increased maternal age and membership of ethnic groups with a high background incidence of type 2 diabetes. GDM most commonly occurs after the middle of the second trimester and can be detected by appropriate screening tests, especially in those at high risk. Perinatal morbidity in GDM increases with increasing maternal hyperglycemia. Much of the pregnancy-related morbidity of GDM is associated with delivering a large-for-gestational-age infant. Women with GDM consistently have increased Cesarian section rates, although this may be reduced by intensive management of maternal hyperglycemia. Sequential ultrasound estimations of fetal growth and abdominal circumference help to identify features of inappropriate fetal growth and inform decisions about the need for intensive blood glucose control. The majority of mothers with GDM can be managed by diet alone. Input from a dietician is mandatory. Care recommendations from Diabetes UK state that blood glucose monitoring should be performed and if pre-prandial levels exceed 6.0 mmol/l (108 mg/dl) insulin treatment should be considered. Insulin dose should be adjusted to achieve pre-prandial levels of 4.0–6.0 mmol/l (72–108 mg/dl).

Many studies have indicated the advantage of controlling post-prandial plasma glucose levels to achieve a good outcome. The American Diabetes Association recommends that insulin therapy should be considered if, on two or more occasions within a 1–2 week interval, dietary management does not maintain fasting plasma glucose below 5.8 mmol/l (105 mg/dl) and/or the 2-hour post-prandial glucose below 6.7 mmol/l (120 mg/dl).

There has long been controversy over the importance of treating GDM. A large NIH-funded multinational study (the Hyperglycemia and Adverse Pregnancy Outcome Study, HAPO) which aims to define the glycemic thresholds during a 75 g OGTT that are associated with an adverse pregnancy outcome should help resolve this dilemma. Recently, a large Australian study examined whether treatment of women with gestational diabetes reduced the risk of perinatal complications. The rate of serious perinatal complications was found to be significantly lower among the infants of the women in the actively treated group with the conclusion that treatment of GDM did indeed reduce serious perinatal morbidity and may also improve the woman's health-related quality of life. On the basis of this research, this view was supported by an editorial in the *New England Journal of Medicine*, although undoubtedly several issues remain, not least of which is the blood glucose level that should trigger active intervention.

The importance of GDM to the mother is that it identifies her as having a metabolic susceptibility for the subsequent development of type 2 diabetes. There is a variable rate of progression to diabetes, with up to 50% of women from ethnic minority groups progressing to diabetes within 5 years of a GDM pregnancy, although this is lower in Caucasian women. There is also an increased risk of cardiovascular disease and such women need to be advised about the benefit of weight loss, exercise and smoking cessation. All women with GDM should have an OGTT 6 weeks after delivery and the results interpreted according to WHO or ADA criteria.

BIBLIOGRAPHY

American Diabetes Association. Gestational diabetes. Diabetes Care 2000; 23 (Suppl 1): S77–9

Crowther CA, Hiller JE, Moss JR, et al. Effect of treatment of gestational diabetes mellitus on pregnancy outcomes. N Engl J Med 2005; 352: 2477–86

Drury IM, Greene AT, Stronge JM. Pregnancy complicated by clinical diabetes mellitus. A study of 600 pregnancies. Obstet Gynecol 1977; 49: 519–22

Greene MF, Solomon CG. Gestational diabetes mellitus – time to treat. N Engl J Med 2005; 352: 2544–6

HAPO Study Cooperative Research Group. The Hyperglycemia and Adverse Pregnancy Outcome (HAPO) Study. Int J Gynaecol Obstet 2002; 78: 69–77

Lowy C. Beard RW, Goldschmidt J. The UK diabetic pregnancy survey. Acta Endocrinol 1986; 277 (Suppl): 86–9

Metzger BE, Coustan DR. Summary and recommendations of the Fourth International Workshop-Conference on Gestational Diabetes Mellitus. Diabetes Care 1998; 21 (Suppl 2): B161–7

Pendersen J. The Pregnant Diabetic and her Newborn. Copenhagen: Munksgaard, 1977

Solomon CG, Willett WC, Rich-Edwards J, et al. Variability in diagnostic evaluation and criteria for gestational diabetes. Diabetes Care 1996; 19: 12–16

Sutherland HW, Stowers JM, eds. Carbohydrate Metabolism in Pregnancy and the Newborn. Edinburgh: Churchill Livingstone, 1984

Williams CB, Iqbal S, Zawacki CM, et al. Effect of selective screening for gestational diabetes. Diabetes Care 1999; 22: 418–21

10 Living with diabetes

Diabetes mellitus, like any chronic medical condition, impacts on quality of life. In one study, at the time of diagnosis of type 1 diabetes, 36% of children exhibited significant psychologic distress. Remarkably, however, in 93% this had completely abated 9 months after diagnosis. Not surprisingly, the parents of newly diagnosed children also experience psychologic upset of a temporary nature, more prominent in mothers. Although not established, adults with new-onset type 1 diabetes probably have similar temporary psychologic responses; however, there is apparently little psychologic morbidity in adults associated with the diagnosis of type 2 diabetes.

Depression is twice as common in adults with type 1 and type 2 diabetes than in a control population and, interestingly, depression commonly precedes the diagnosis in type 2 patients. The course of depression in diabetes may be particularly chronic and severe.

The diagnosis of diabetes has effects on other aspects of the diabetic patient's life. In most developed countries, drivers with diabetes have a statutory requirement to declare their diabetes to the national licensing authority. Furthermore, failure to do so may invalidate motor insurance policies. Following declaration of the diagnosis of diabetes, a driving license is issued for a maximum of 3 years in the UK, but is renewable at no cost following completion of a medical questionnaire. If a patient reports a medical problem that may affect safe driving then the licensing authority will solicit more detailed medical reports. Most countries impose limitations on the issue of vocational licenses (heavy goods vehicles, passenger carrying vehicles) to insulin-treated diabetic drivers.

Diabetic individuals treated with insulin or sulfonylureas are not permitted to fly commercial aircraft or to work as air-traffic controllers.

Diabetic patients may experience difficulties with employment. Statutory or company policy may disbar them from certain occupations and these include train drivers, the armed forces, off-shore oil-rig work, etc. Furthermore, even when there is no risk due to possible hypoglycemia, discrimination by employers may affect hiring practices leading to loss of self-esteem and earning ability, and impacting on the patient's ability to support a family and their future quality of life.

Insurance may also prove to pose problems for individuals with diabetes. Insurance companies may refuse to accept diabetic applicants for life insurance or impose restrictions or inflated premiums. More favorable insurance terms may be provided by approved brokers recommended by national diabetes associations.

There are many other areas in life where having diabetes may cause difficulties and they include travel overseas, insurance and medical care abroad, exposure to unusual foods and drinks in different countries and the effect of intercurrent illness and sport on day-to-day blood glucose control.

BIBLIOGRAPHY

Kovacs M, Goldston D, Obrosky DS, Bonar LK. Psychiatric disorders in youths with IDDM: rates and risk factors. Diabetes Care 1997; 20: 36–44

11 Future developments in diabetes

Research activity in the field of diabetes has increased greatly in recent years. People with diabetes would want this to translate into more effective treatment of diabetes and its complications. Patients with type 1 diabetes would like to be freed from the need to self-inject with insulin. Pancreatic and islet-cell transplantation can achieve this; however, it is unlikely that these techniques will find widespread application in the immediate future. It may prove possible to generate mature β-cells from embryonic stem cells, but many issues need to be resolved before cells derived by these methods can be used in human transplantation. Although experimental gene therapy (with transfer of DNA to somatic cells) has shown promising results, no proposed gene therapy model for the treatment or prevention of diabetes has reached the stage of clinical testing. Technological developments to produce implantable insulin pumps with continuous glucose sensing continue, but are not sufficiently advanced to allow wide uptake. Until sufficient progress in these areas has been achieved, it is likely that most progress will be made through the development of new pharmaceutical products to treat the hyperglycemia of diabetes. Such activity is burgeoning. New insulin analogs continue to appear. Several devices allowing the pulmonary delivery of inhaled insulin have already been developed. Inhaled insulin treatment is being actively investigated as an alternative non-invasive method of insulin delivery and many studies have already attested to its effectiveness in achieving tight glycemic control in both type 1 and type 2 diabetes. Oral insulins have also been developed but are only at a preliminary level of investigation. Perhaps the most exciting

potential therapy area lies in the discovery and evaluation of new drugs to treat type 2 diabetes. Insulin secretion can be stimulated by the incretin gut hormones glucagon-like peptide-1 (GLP-1) and glucose-dependent insulinotropic polypeptide (GIP) without leading to hypoglycemia. Stable analogs of these incretins have been developed with a longer half-life. Such an analog, exenatide, Byetta® Amylin pharmaceuticals (exendin-4), when injected subcutaneously has been shown to reduce HbA_{1c} in patients with type 2 diabetes failing to achieve glycemic control on maximal doses of either metformin alone or metformin/sulfonylurea combination. Inhibitors of dipeptidyl peptidase-IV (DPP-IV) which degrades GLP-1 have also been developed and have reached an advanced stage of clinical trial. Amylin, a polypeptide synthesized by the islet β-cells and co-secreted with insulin, appears to act centrally to induce satiety, slow gastric emptying and suppress pancreatic glucagon secretion. Pramlintide is a soluble analog of amylin with amylin-like effects which last for about 3 hours after subcutaneous administration prior to a meal. It has been launched in the USA as Symlin®, Amylin pharmaceuticals and is licensed in both type 1 and 2 diabetes as an adjunct to meal-time insulin therapy in those who have failed to achieve desired glucose control despite optimal insulin therapy. One of its main advantages is that it is not associated with weight gain. Other exciting drugs in development are dual peroxisome proliferator-activated receptor (PPAR)α and γ agonists, which may treat both hyperglycemia and dyslipidemia, and rimonabant which acts on the endocannabinoid system. Endocannabinoids act on cannabinoid type 1 (CB$_1$) and type 2 (CB$_2$) receptors. The endocannabinoid system plays a key role in the regulation of energy balance and fat accumulation and overactivity of the system is associated with increased food intake and fat accumulation. Rimonabant acts as a selective CB$_1$ blocker inducing weight loss, reducing triglyceride levels and improving glucose tolerance. It presents a novel tool to reduce cardiovascular risk factors of the metabolic syndrome including dyslipidemia and type 2 diabetes (as well as nicotine dependence). Rimonabant (Acomplia®, Sanofi-Aventis), has already obtained regulatory approval as an adjunct to diet and exercise for the treatment of obese patients or overweight patients with associated risk factors.

Thus, many potentially useful pharmacologic agents are currently being investigated with some at a late stage of clinical trial. The hope is that such advances will feed through to real clinical benefit for patients with diabetes.

BIBLIOGRAPHY

Day C. Amylin analogue as an antidiabetic agent. Br J Diabetes Vasc Dis 2005; 5: 151–4

DeFronzo RA, Ratner RE, Han J, et al. Effects of exenatide (exendin-4) on glycemic control and weight over 30 weeks in metformin-treated patients with type 2 diabetes. Diabetes Care 2005; 28: 1092–100

Finer N, Pagotto U. The endocannabinoid system: a new therapeutic target for cardiovascular risk factor management. Br J Diabetes Vasc Dis 2005; 5: 121–4

Green BD, Irwin N, Gault VA, et al. Development and therapeutic potential of incretin hormone analogues for type 2 diabetes. Br J Diabetes Vasc Dis 2005; 5: 134–40

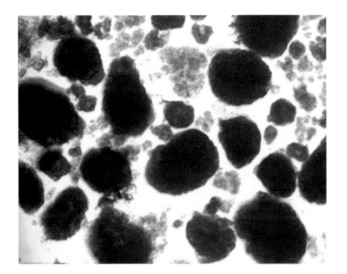

Figure 153 Intact islet cells ready for islet cell transplantation. The islets are isolated from donated human pancreas, suspended during partial digestion and centrifuged in a cooled centrifuge. The retrieval of good quality islets from donor pancreases is critical to the success of islet cell transplantation

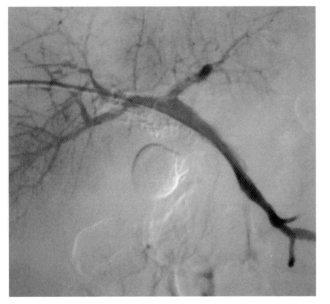

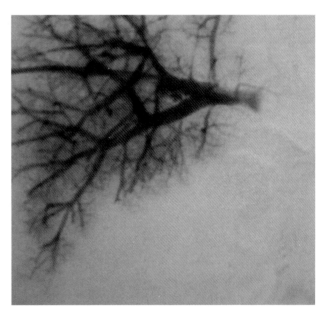

Figure 154 Portal venogram showing the hepatic portal vein prior to administration of isolated human islets. In the Edmonton protocol, an adequate mass of freshly isolated islets are embolized for transplantation into the liver through a small catheter placed into the main portal vein. Novel immunosuppressive regimens, as outlined in the text, have led to an increased success rate of this experimental mode of therapy of diabetes

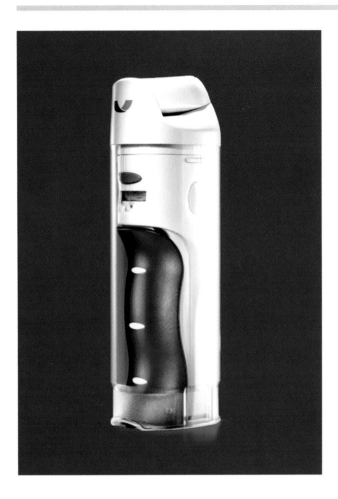

Figure 155 Several pharmaceutical companies have developed inhaled short-acting insulin preparations using different technology and inhalation devices. One such product, Exubera® (Pfizer) has recently been granted marketing authorization by the European Commission and will shortly be available on prescription. Clinical studies have attested to an efficiency of inhaled insulin to control daytime blood glucose levels comparable to that of soluble insulin. Regulatory agencies have expressed concern about long-term pulmonary safety

Index

acanthosis nigricans 77, 104
acromegaly 2, 18
acute complications of DM 63–7
Addison's disease 18
adenovirus 12
adhesive capsulitis, shoulder 78
alcohol 33, 63
alprostadil (prostaglandin E_1) 76, 90, 91
American Diabetes Association (ADA)
    diagnostic criteria 1–2, 14
    etiologic classification 6
    exercise guidelines 34
    GDM criteria 112, 113
    HbA_{1c} target 38
    hyperlipidemia screening recommendations 110
    Working Group on the Prevention of Diabetes
        recommendations 14
amputation, lower-limb 73, 74
amylin 11, 117
angiotensin II receptor antagonist 73
angiotensin-converting enzyme (ACE) inhibitor 70,
    73–4
apomorphine 76
arthropathy
    Charcot's 74, 93, 94
    cheiroarthropathy 77–8, 106
atheromatous lesions 73
atorvastatin 109, 110

B lymphocytes 10
bacterial infection, skin 105
Bacteroides spp. 74
balanitis 104
Banting, Frederick 4
becaplermin 95

bendrofluazide 74
Best, Charles H. 4
beta-blockers 74
bezafibrate 110
blood glucose 36–7
    monitoring systems 37, 56, 117
    plasma profile
        'glucose excursions' 55
        insulin injections 49, 50
        non-diabetic 49
        stable control 55
    self-monitoring technique 53
    subcutaneously implanted continuous monitoring
        system 37, 56, 117
bovine serum albumin 10
'brittle' diabetics 38
bullae 77, 103

calcium-channel blockers 74
calorie restriction 34
candidiasis 104
carbohydrates, dietary management of type 1 DM 33
cardiovascular disease 73
    recurrent coronary heart disease (CHD) events 73
carpal tunnel syndrome 72
β-cells, pancreatic
    autoimmune destruction 10
    dysfunction 10–12
    monogenetic defects 2, 9
    stem cell generated 117
    viral infection 9–10
Charcot's arthropathy 74, 93, 94
cheiroarthropathy 77–8, 106
children and adolescents
    childhood obesity 21

childhood type 2 diabetes 2
    continuous subcutaneous insulin infusion (CSII) 60
    emotional problems 59
    hypoglycemia 59
    insulin requirements 59–60
    macrosomic babies 108, 111
    puberty 60
    treatment 59–60
cholesterol 33, 109
Cholesterol and Recurrent Events Trial (CARE) 109
chronic complications of DM 69–108
cirrhosis 76–7
classification of DM 2–3, 6
Collaborative Atorvastatin Diabetes Study (CARDS)
        109
coma, hyperosmolar non-ketoacidotic 67
continuous ambulatory peritoneal dialysis (CAPD) 71
continuous subcutaneous insulin infusion (CSII) 60
Coxsackie B virus 10, 12
creatinine level 70–1, 112
Cushing's syndrome 2, 17
cystic fibrosis 2, 28
cytomegalovirus 10, 12

Da Qing study, China 14
depression 115
dermopathy 77, 102
Diabetes Control and Complications Trial (DCCT),
        USA 35, 37, 63, 69
diabetes mellitus (DM), definition 1
Diabetes Prevention Program, USA 14
diabetes specialist nurses (DSNs) 37, 61
Diabetes UK, GDM recommendations 112
'diabetic foods' 33
diagnostic criteria of DM 1–2, 7
dialysis 71
diazoxide 2
dietary advice 56, 57
DIGAMI study 73
dipeptidyl peptidase-IV (DPP-IV) inhibitor 117
Dose Adjustment for Normal Eating (DAFNE) program
        37–8
Down's syndrome 2, 12
doxazosin 74
driving licence, UK 115
drug treatment
    dose range, distribution and half-life 58
    type 2 diabetes 39–40
Dupuytren's contracture 78, 107
dyslipidemia 109–10

endocannabinoid system 117–18
entrapment syndrome 72, 87
environmental factors
    for children and adolescents 59–60
    viral infection 9, 10, 12, 30
Epstein–Barr virus 10
erectile dysfunction (ED)
    causes 75
    hypogonadism 76
    treatment 76, 89
    vacuum pump system 76, 88
    vasoactive drug
        injection 76, 90
        transurethral application 76, 90
eruptive xanthomata 77, 105, 106
Escherichia coli 44
European Diabetes Project Group, HbA$_{1c}$ target 38
European Nicotinamide Diabetes Intervention Trial
        (ENDIT) 13
exenatide 117
exercise 34
    and insulin sensitivity 34
eye disorders
    DIDMOAD syndrome 80
    laser photocoagulation 84
    maculopathy 82
    normal fundus 80
    ophthalmology referral 85
    retinal detachment 82
    retinopathy 69–70, 80–5
    thromboneovascular glaucoma 84
    triamcinolone therapy 82
    vitreous hemorrhage 85
ezetimibe 110

fasting plasma glucose (FGP) concentration 1
fat intake 33, 34
fenofibrate 110
fibrates 110
fiber, dietary 33
fibrocalculous pancreatopathy 2
Finnish Diabetes Prevention Study 14, 71
foot disorders
    burn injuries 88
    callus 74
    Charcot's arthropathy 74, 93, 94
    deep infection 74, 93
    digital arterial calcification 75, 97, 98
    gangrene 96, 97
    osteomyelitis 74, 75, 94

treatment 75, 95
ulcer 74, 92, 95
weight-bearing reduction 95
future developments
β-cells, stem cell generated 117
continuous glucose monitoring 117
inhaled insulin delivery 117, 119
insulin pumps 117
islet cell transplantation 117
oral insulin delivery 117
pancreatic transplantation 117
pharmaceutical products 117–18

gastric neurostimulator (GES) system 88
gemfibrozil 77, 109, 110
genes
DBQ1 9
glucokinase 12
INS (insulin gene) 9
genetic loci
7p (glucokinase) 12
11p5.5 (IDDM2) 9
geographic variation of DM 1, 3
gestational diabetes mellitus (GDM) 2, 14, 112
ADA recommendations 112, 113
Cesarian section rates 112
Diabetes UK recommendations 112
HAPO study 113
O'Sullivan–Mahan criteria (USA) 2
WHO criteria 2, 112, 113
see also pregnancy
glitazones 14, 39–40, 41, 77
glomerulopathy 91
glucagon-like peptide-1 (GLP-1) 11, 117
glucocorticoids 2
glucose
metabolism, brain 66
tolerance, impaired 2, 3, 11, 14
see also blood glucose
glucose-dependent insulinotropic polypeptide (GIP)
11, 117
α-glucosidase inhibitors 39
glucotoxicity 11
glutamic acid decarboxylase (GAD) antibodies 10
gluten 10
glycemic control 38, 70
granuloma annulare 102

health-care costs 1
Heart Outcomes Prevention Evaluation Study (HOPE
study) 74
hemochromatosis 2, 19, 29
hemoglobin (HbA$_{1c}$) 34

in pregnancy 111
targets 38
hepatic nuclear factors (HFNs) 2, 11–12
hepatic portal vein, isolated islet administration 119
high-density lipoprotein (HDL) 109
human leukocyte antigen (HLA) 9
HLA antigens 9
hydroxymethylglutaryl-coenzyme A reductase inhibitor
109–10
hyperbaric oxygen 75
hyperglycemia 11
in pregnancy 111
sugars 33
in surgery 61
symptoms 1
Hyperglycemic Adverse Pregnancy Outcome (HAPO)
study 113
hyperinsulinemia 11, 77
hyperlipidemia 71, 109–10
hyperosmolar non-ketoacidotic coma 67
hypertension 70–1, 73–4
hypertriglyceridemia 109
hypoglycemia 33–7, 63, 65
brain glucose metabolism 66
children and adolescents 59
hypoglycemia-induced cardiac dysrhythmia 63
neonatal 111
in surgery 61
symptoms 63
hypoinsulinemia 34
fetal 111

IDDM1 9
IDDM2 9
impaired fasting glucose (IFG) 2
impaired glucose tolerance (IGT) 2, 3, 11, 14
indapamide 74
insulin
absorption rate, factors affecting 50
administration sites 48
biosynthesis 44
biphasic response to glucose 22
crystals 43
deficiency, biochemical consequences 23
discovery of 4
impaired secretion 10
infuser 51, 117
inhalation delivery system 117, 119
injection technique 49
lipid hypertrophy 52, 53
lipoatrophy 52
longer-acting 35, 40
oral delivery 117

pens 35, 46–7
plasma profile, non-diabetic 49
proinsulin, protein sequence 43
rapid-acting 35
requirements, children and adolescents 59–60
resistance 2, 10–12
syringes 46
insulin analogs and formulations 45
insulin aspart 35, 60
insulin detemir 35–6, 40
insulin glargine 35–6, 40
insulin glulisine 35
insulin lispro 35, 60
NPH (isophane) 35, 40
porcine insulin 36
protamine retarded 60
insulin autoantibodies (IAA) 10
insulin promoter factor-1 11
insulin regimes
basal-bolus 35–6
continuous subcutaneous insulin infusion (CSII) 36, 60
twice-daily 35
insulin resistance syndrome 2, 10–12
definition 12
insulin-dependent diabetes mellitus (IDDM) see type 1 diabetes
insulin-like growth factor (IGF)-1 77
insulinoma 25
insulitis 10
insurance issues 115
interferon (IFN)γ 10
interleukin (IL)-2 10
islet of Langerhans
Coxsackie B viral infection (LM) 30
cystic fibrosis, pancreas (LM) 28
glucagon immunostained (LM) 24
hemochromatosis, hemosiderin deposits (LM) 29
insulin immunostained (LM) 24
insulin storage granules (EM) 25
insulitis hyperexpression (LM) 28
normal pancreas (EM) 25
normal pancreas (LM) 24
somatostatin immunostained 25
type 1 DM
β-cells (LM) 26
β-cell loss (LM) 27
infiltrate (LM) 26
lymphocyte infiltration (LM) 27
type 2 DM
amyloid deposition (LM) 29
islet amyloid polypeptide (IAPP) 11
islet cell antibodies (ICA) 10, 28

islet cell transplantation 41, 117, 119

jaundice, neonatal 111

ketoacidosis 64
biomechanical features 66
causes of death 67
ketosis, in surgery 61
Klinefelter's syndrome 2, 12, 19

laser photocoagulation 70, 84
latent autoimmune diabetes in adults (LADA) 2
late-onset diabetes mellitus 2
immune-mediated type 1 2
lifestyle change 14
lipid hypertrophy 52, 53
liver
cirrhosis 76–7
glucose output 11
glucose production 22
hepatic nuclear factors (HFNs) 2, 11–12
hepatic portal vein, isolated islet administration 119
low-density lipoprotein (LDL) 109–10

macrophages 10
macrosomic babies 108, 111
maculopathy 69–70
maggot debridement, ulcer 75
major histocompatibility complex (MHC) 9
antigens 10
male excess, type 1 1
malignant otitis externa 105
maturity-onset diabetes of the young (MODY) 2, 11–12
symptoms 12
meglitinides 39
metabolic syndrome see insulin resistance syndrome
metformin 39, 41, 77
migratory necrolytic erythema 77, 103
monitoring systems, blood glucose 37, 56, 117
mumps 10, 12
myotonic dystrophy 20

National Institute of Diabetes and Digestive and Kidney Diseases (NIDDK), USA trials 13
necrobiosis lipoidica diabeticorum 77, 101
nephropathy 70–1
neurogenic differentiation factor (NEUROD) 1 11
neuropathy
acute 72
autonomic 72–3, 87
chronic insidious sensory 72
classification 86

mononeuropathy 72
  pathogenesis 71–2
  prevalence 71
  proximal motor 72
  third cranial nerve palsy 87
  treatment 73
  ulnar 87
nitrosamines 10
non-alcoholic steatohepatitis (NASH) 76–7
non-insulin-dependent diabetes mellitus (NIDDM) *see* type 2 diabetes

obesity
  body mass index (BMI) 12, 16
  childhood 21
  energy expenditure 13
  epidemic 12
  food consumption 12
  sequelae 13
oral glucose tolerance test (OGTT) 1–2, 112
orlistat 34, 40
osteomyelitis 74, 75, 94, 99
  foot 74, 75, 94
  spinal 99
osteoporosis 94, 99

pancreas
  calcification 31
  cancer 2
  cancer (CT scan) 31
  hemochromatosis 29
  pancreatic duct, normal 30
  transplantation 41–2, 117
  trauma 2
  see also β-cell; islet of Langerhans
pancreatectomy 2
pancreatitis 2
patient education 37–8
peripheral vascular disease 73, 74, 97, 98
peroxisome proliferator-activated receptors (PPAR)
  agonists 40, 110, 117
pheochromocytoma 2
phosphodiesterase inhibitors 76
plasminogen activator inhibitor type 1 (PAI-1) 73
platelet-derived growth factor 75
polycythemia, neonatal 111
Prader–Willi syndrome 16
pramlintide 117
prandial glucose regulators 39
pravastatin 110
pregnancy 2, 111–13
  Caesarean section rates 111–12
  haemoglobin (HbA$_{1c}$) 111

insulin regimes 111–12
  neonatal problems 112
  perinatal problems 111
  pre-eclampsia 112
  ultrasound scans 112
  see also gestational diabetes mellitus (GDM)
prevention trials, pharmacological
  ACT NOW (pioglitazone) 14
  DREAM (ramipril and rosiglitazone) 14
  NAVIGATOR (nateglinide and valsartan) 14
  ORIGIN (insulin glargine) 14
proteinuria 70
puberty 60
pulmonary delivery, inhaled insulin delivery 117

quality of life issues 115

Rabson–Mendenhall syndrome 21
random plasma glucose concentration 1
Reaven's syndrome *see* insulin resistance syndrome
α-receptor blockers 74
relative insulin deficiency 2
renal
  artery stenosis 73
  failure 71, 92
  glomerulopathy 91
  transplantation 71
retinopathy 69–70, 80–5
  background 80
  end-stage 84
  exudative 82
  peripheral proliferative 83
  serious 81
  severe 81
rimonabant 118
rosuvastatin 110
rubella, congenital 12

Scandinavian Simvastatin Survival Study (4S Trial) 109
sibutramine 40
sildenafil 76, 89
simvastatin 109, 110
skin disorders 77, 100
  acanthosis nigricans 77, 104
  balanitis 104
  bullae 77, 103
  candidiasis 104
  dermopathy 77, 102
  eruptive xanthomata 77, 105, 106
  granuloma annulare 102
  migratory necrolytic erythema 77, 103
  necrobiosis lipoidica diabeticorum 77, 101
  severe bacterial infection 105

uncommon 77
vitiligo 77, 100
skin graft
bi-layered bioengineered skin substitute 75
cultured human dermis 75
smoking 34
sodium restriction 33
Staphylococcus aureus 74
statin therapy 109–10
lipid-lowering combination therapy
statin/ezetimibe 109–10
statin/fibrate 109–10
steatohepatitis 76–7
Streptococcus pyogenes 74
Study to Prevent Non-Insulin Dependent Diabetes
(STOP-NIDDM) Trial, multinational 14
subcutaneously implanted continuous monitoring
system, blood glucose 37, 56, 117
sulfonylureas 39, 41, 63
surgery 61–2
insulin regimens 62
perioperative complications 61
postoperative infection 61
syndrome X *see* insulin resistance syndrome

T lymphocytes 9–10
tachycardia 73
tadalafil 76
thiazide 2
thiazolidinediones 14, 39–40
transplantation
islet cell 41, 117, 119
renal 71
simultaneous pancreas-kidney transplants (SPKs)
41–2
whole-pancreas 41, 117
triglycerides 109–10
truncal radiculopathy 72
tumor necrosis factor (TNF)-α 10
Turner's syndrome 2, 12, 20
type 1 diabetes
classification 2–3
dietary advice 57
epidemiology 3
ethnic variation 9
incidence 1
male excess 1, 3

pathogenesis 9–10
pre-insulin treatment 4
prevention 13
surgery 61
treatment
dietary 33
insulin 35–6
viral associations 30
type 2 diabetes
childhood 2
classification 2–3
dietary advice 57
dietary treatment 34
epidemiology 3
incidence 1
pathogenesis 10–11
prevention 13–14
surgery 62
treatment
drugs 39–40
HbA$_{1c}$ targets 38
insulin 40

United Kingdom Prospective Diabetes Study (UKPDS)
38, 69
Blood Pressure Control Study 74
HbA$_{1c}$ target 38
ursodeoxycholic acid 77

vardenafil 76
very-low-density lipoprotein (VLDL) 109
Veterans Affairs HDL Intervention Trial (VA-HIT) 109
viral associations
adenovirus 12
β-cells, viral infection 9–10
Coxsackie B virus 10, 12
cytomegalovirus 10, 12
Epstein–Barr virus 10
type 1 diabetes 30
vitiligo 77, 100

weight loss 14, 34
Wolfram's syndrome 12
World Health Organization (WHO)
diagnostic criteria 1
GDM criteria 112, 113